ALSO BY JEFFREY A. FISHER, M.D.

The Chromium Program
Rx 2000

Contents

THE PLAGUE MAKERS

HOW WE ARE CREATING

CATASTROPHIC NEW EPIDEMICS—

AND WHAT WE MUST DO

TO AVERT THEM

JEFFREY A. FISHER, M.D.

SIMON & SCHUSTER

NEW YORK   LONDON   TORONTO   SYDNEY   TOKYO   SINGAPORE

SIMON & SCHUSTER
Rockefeller Center
1230 Avenue of the Americas
New York, New York 10020

Designed by Irving Perkins Associates
Manufactured in the United States of America

10   9   8   7   6   5   4   3   2   1

Library of Congress Cataloging-in-Publication Data
Fisher, Jeffrey A., date
     The plague makers : how we are creating catastrophic new
epidemics—and what we must do to avert them / Jeffrey A. Fisher.
          p.   cm.
     Includes bibliographical references.
     1. Antibiotics—Side effects.   2. Drug resistance in
microorganisms.   3. Nosocomial infections.   I. Title.
RM267.F53   1994
615′.329—dc20   93-45761
                                                                      CIP

ISBN: 0-671-79156-7

PART ONE

THE DIMENSIONS OF THE THREAT

CHAPTER 1

Prelude to Disaster

A fifty-year-old businessman, in good health, takes the late-evening shuttle from La Guardia Airport in New York to Boston, where he has several appointments the next day. Shortly after checking into his hotel, he notices he has a stuffy nose and scratchy throat. What he assumes is a mild cold becomes more severe during the night: a 102-degree fever, chills and a dry cough. The next morning, now thinking he has the flu, he cancels all his appointments and flies back to New York. Three days later, despite receiving massive doses of a cephalosporin antibiotic, he dies in the hospital of a devastating pneumonia.

A twenty-eight-year-old basketball player has a routine blood test when he applies for a large life insurance policy. The following week, his physician informs him that he is HIV-positive. He assures him, however, that all other biochemical parameters are normal and that he is still in good health. He does not have AIDS and is encouraged to continue playing basketball. A month later, while on the road, he feels a little tired. He reaches into his equipment bag for some antibiotics he always carries with him, and which he uses routinely, on a doctor's prescription, to ward off colds and other minor infections. Within a day he feels better. Three months later, he is diagnosed with AIDS and the following year he is dead.

❖   ❖   ❖

A young mother notices that her three-year-old daughter seems restless and feverish and is constantly pulling at her ear. The pediatrician diagnoses a middle-ear infection and prescribes the antibiotic amoxicillin, which he says should clear up the problem in a few days. The child, however, gets worse. The fever goes higher, she begins vomiting and her neck becomes stiff. She is rushed to the hospital emergency room in the middle of the night where a spinal tap is performed and acute bacterial meningitis is diagnosed. Despite the administration of intravenous antibiotics, she dies the next morning.

A forty-four-year-old physician with a history of recurrent bladder infections experiences burning on urination, this time accompanied by blood in the urine, a high fever and pain in her right flank. She correctly self-diagnoses that she has pyelonephritis, a serious kidney infection, and calls her friend, a kidney specialist. He says what she dreads: she must be admitted to the hospital for intravenous antibiotics.

Why should physicians, for whom the sights, sounds and smells of the hospital are part of their everyday routine, be afraid to be patients? It is simply because, far more than anyone else, they are aware of the danger lurking there. They know too well that in those gleaming, high-tech institutions, where medical miracles are performed every day, roam the ghosts from the wards of the past, from a time we thought we'd never have to see again. They know that although in the 1990s the typical hospital patient is admitted with an organic disease such as cancer, heart disease, stroke or diabetic complications, the pendulum has incredibly begun to swing back to the 1930s. They know that hospitals are in jeopardy of once again being overwhelmed with untreatable infectious diseases such as pneumonia, tuberculosis, meningitis, typhoid fever and dysentery. And they know that just by being in a hospital they are at risk of contracting one of these deadly illnesses.

Sixty years ago infectious diseases were the main cause of pain and death because we had so little to combat them. This was before the discovery of antibiotic drugs. Today a physician has countless numbers of antibiotics to choose from. In 1992, there were 420 anti-infective products on the United States market. Yet, despite this impressive armamentarium, every day patients die of untreatable infections in hospitals in New York, London, Paris, Tokyo and Barcelona. The shocking case of the Muppets' creator, Jim Henson, who died suddenly a few years ago in a New York hospital from a fulminant case of pneumonia, was not an anomaly but a harbinger.

We seem to have come full cycle. The infections that are cutting a wide swath through our hospitals today are completely resistant to the antibiotics we have come to blindly rely on. As a result physicians are once again helpless. Just as in the preantibiotic era, they can only stand by, console the family and pray for miracles. Before the advent of antibiotics we had no therapeutic options. Today, many experts believe we've just about exhausted them.

Hospitals aren't the only place where danger waits. Bacteria that could be responsible for the new epidemics of antibiotic-resistant pneumonia, meningitis and a host of other infections can be transmitted by casual contact in a shopping mall or a movie theater. Fatalities from a wide range of infectious diseases are occurring today with alarming frequency throughout the world. And they signal a potential for disaster that could involve millions of people in the next decade or even sooner. We are standing on the brink of a catastrophe. And if nothing is done to prevent it, we will suffer a new plague of infectious diseases more devastating than any we have experienced in the past.

The seeds of the crisis were sown a long time ago, paradoxically the moment antibiotics were introduced to the world. In fact, the notion that therapy for infectious diseases would be a double-edged sword was actually recognized nearly one hundred years ago, long before antibiotics were known. The German Nobel laureate Paul Ehrlich, father of immunology and the specific therapy of infectious disease, noted that syphilis bacteria could develop resistance to the arsenic-derived compound he had formulated. Salvarsan, the name of Dr. Ehrlich's drug, was not an antibiotic, and Dr. Ehrlich didn't know exactly how the resistance developed, but the biochemical mechanism was similar to what would later be demonstrated with antibiotics.

While there are reports of scientists in Germany and England in the late nineteenth and early twentieth centuries finding molds with antibacterial properties, the modern antibiotic era is associated with only one name. In 1928, Sir Alexander Fleming serendipitously discovered the antibacterial properties of the bread mold extract penicillin. But being a pure laboratory scientist Fleming apparently did not initially consider the remarkable therapeutic value of his finding. It would be almost fifteen years before two Oxford scientists, Howard Florey and Ernst B. Chain, tested and proved the value of penicillin in humans. The mass production of penicillin followed within a few years. This, along with the discovery of sulfa drugs by Gerhard Domagk in Germany in the 1930s, of streptomycin by Rutgers University soil microbiologist Selman Waksman, and cephalosporin by Giuseppe Brotzu in the mid-1940s, began the antibiotic era and revolutionized the practice of medicine.

These were heady times for physicians. They finally had something they could use to slay the bacterial dragons that had been a scourge for centuries and had, at several times in the course of history, all but wiped out whole populations. Doctors began using the new wonder drugs, the "magic bullets" that Ehrlich had sought but never found, for virtually everything. And they were almost universally successful. Survival rates for the dreaded pneumonia, for example, called in 1901 the "captain of the men of death" by world-famous physician Sir William Osler, increased dramatically from less than 20 percent in 1937 to 85 percent by 1964. As Walsh McDermott described in a 1982 article in the *Johns Hopkins Medical Journal*, the introduction of antibiotics into medical practice "heralded the opening of an era in which literally millions of people—children, adults and the elderly, all slated for early death or invalidism—were spared." The family doctor became a hero.

The discovery of antibiotics still ranks as one of the greatest medical achievements of the twentieth century. And new ways of effectively using them are still being discovered. As recently as 1992, for example, it was shown that some ulcers, for decades thought to be the result of excess stomach acid, were instead almost certainly caused by a common type of bacteria called *Helicobacter* and could in turn be cured by antibiotics. There were other stunning medical advances perfected during the 1930s and 1940s. But it was antimicrobial therapy that was the real artillery, providing physicians with the ability to prevent some infections, to cure others, and to curtail the transmission of diseases.

It's really not difficult to understand why no one stopped to heed the danger signs that were pointed out. In Fleming's original 1929 paper in the *British Journal of Experimental Pathology* he noted that, while penicillin was remarkably effective in inhibiting the growth of staphylococci in the laboratory, it was completely ineffective against other forms of bacteria called *B. coli* (now referred to as *E. coli*). Eleven years later, while working with penicillin at Oxford, Ernst B. Chain, along with his colleague Edward P. Abraham, isolated an enzyme from the *B. coli* that was able to destroy penicillin, giving biochemical credibility to Fleming's observation.

On the basis of these laboratory studies, quiet cautions began to be issued to physicians. As early as 1942, even before penicillin began to be used commercially, Fleming alerted the medical profession that staphylococci might find a way to develop the resistance he had seen in the *B. coli* bacteria. Two years later, in 1944, just after penicillin was introduced to the American market, Florey publicly decried the misuse that was already apparent in Britain. Physicians were giving penicillin like candy. Supply couldn't keep up with demand.

Florey had noted that during treatment with penicillin, the inherently resistant *B. coli*, along with other bacteria whose disease-causing potential was unknown, actually increased in number. Most disturbing of all, Florey cited cases where the effectiveness of this newly introduced wonder drug might already be waning. There were clinical examples that required up to eight times the usual starting dose before an infection could be tamed.

But Florey, Fleming, and other sober minds were drowned out by the intoxication of the moment. No one wanted to hear any bad news. Medical Cassandras had no place in the era of miracle drugs.

It wasn't long, though, before their predictions began to come true. Reports of outbreaks of infections difficult or impossible to handle because of bacterial resistance to antibiotics started being reported in medical journals in the 1940s.

This is what is even more disturbing than the gravity of the situation confronting us. Antibiotic resistance hasn't just appeared on the medical landscape. It's been developing for more than fifty years right under our noses, yet we've done virtually nothing to slow it down. Microbiologists and infectious disease experts have been discussing this problem for decades, but mostly among themselves, in hushed tones behind the closed doors of medical meetings or in the scientific literature.

There was a brief period when the discussion got beyond ivory-tower academics; in December 1984, a two-day congressional hearing on antibiotic resistance was conducted by Vice President Albert Gore in his last days as a member of the House of Representatives. Revelatory and striking testimony was taken from several experts, testimony that outlined the multitude of causes and very real and forbidding consequences of antibiotic resistance. But no action was taken. And how many of us were even aware that the hearings took place? It seems strange that this issue quietly died. Perhaps it was because Mr. Gore moved on to the Senate and other concerns, leaving behind no one to carry the ball. Vice President Gore's staff was extremely helpful in providing me with information and material about the 1984 hearings, but the question about why this wasn't followed up was deftly sidestepped no matter whom I asked.

The problem of antibiotic resistance is something that most practicing physicians seem either indifferent to or ignorant about. I remember my microbiology lectures in medical school, where I first learned about the ability of bacteria to develop resistance to antibiotics. The information was delivered almost in passing, as an aside. And the subject never came up again, not during my pediatric internship, when I was using antibiotics every day, and not later as a practicing pathologist, when I was responsible for supervising a microbiology laboratory and chairing the infection control committees in several community hospitals. I would attend national meetings devoted to better performance of these duties, but monitoring and trying to limit antibiotic resistance were never once discussed. Most young physicians—myself included—filed the subject away on a three-by-five card in the back of their mind, alongside the biochemical intermediates of cellular glucose metabolism and the intricate life cycles of obscure tropical parasites we would never face in clinical practice.

How blind we've been can be understood by the following, by no means complete, chronology:

• During the latter part of World War II, there were several serious epidemics of pneumonia in the armed forces caused by beta-hemolytic streptococci. These organisms were highly resistant to the sulfa drug sulfadiazine, the only available antimicrobial agent and a drug to which the streptococci had been thought to be universally sensitive. Curiously, sulfadiazine had been used earlier as part of an extensive prophylactic campaign among the troops to prevent just such epidemics.

• In the mid-1940s, Fleming's forecast became reality when the first strains of *Staphylococcus* resistant to penicillin were described. Today, in excess of 95 percent of *Staphylococcus* worldwide are resistant to penicillin.

• In 1955, a Japanese woman who recently had returned from visiting Hong Kong came down with a stubborn case of dysentery. The causative agent was isolated and identified as a typical dysentery bacterium, *Shigella*. But it was far from an ordinary *Shigella*. This *Shigella* was highly resistant to four antibiotics: sulfa, streptomycin, chloramphenicol and tetracycline.

Although recognized at the time by only a few astute Japanese scientists, this event was a warning of dangerous things to occur in subsequent decades. It was the first time a bacterium had been shown to be multiply resistant to antibiotics. In the next few years the incidence of multiply drug-resistant shigellae in Japan increased, and there were a number of epidemics of intractable dysentery.

• In 1963, there began to be reports of several strains of pneumococci, the most common cause of pneumonia at the time, that were resistant to tetracycline. This was not just a laboratory finding but resulted in several treatment failures and deaths. Shortly thereafter, strains of pneumococci resistant to the antibiotics erythromycin and lincomycin were reported almost simultaneously in England and New York.

• In 1967 from Australia came the first report of pneumococci resistant to penicillin. This was followed in 1971 by a short paper in *The New England Journal of Medicine* which reported a reduced susceptibility to penicillin in carriers and patients with pneumonia in New Guinea. Because penicillin had been used in one area of New Guinea for prophylaxis of pneumonia, concern was expressed that this was responsible for the 25-fold lower than average susceptibility of the pneumococcal bacteria isolated.

• In Iran, within a ten-year period between 1963 and 1973, the strain of *Salmonella* causing epidemics changed from almost 100 percent sensitive to almost 100 percent resistant.

• *Neisseria gonorrhoeae,* the bacterium responsible for gonorrhea, was almost uniformly sensitive to penicillin until 1975, when a few resistant cases were observed in the Philippines. Today, in excess of 90 percent of *Neisseria gonorrhoeae* in the Philippines and Thailand is resistant to penicillin and almost 50 percent in India, Africa, Japan, western Europe and the United States.

• Resistance of the bacterium *Hemophilus influenzae*—the most common cause of serious ear infections and meningitis in children younger than five years old—to the antibiotic ampicillin didn't begin to show up at all until 1974. When first observed, the resistance was found in only about 4 percent of blood and spinal fluid samples in the United States, but by 1982 it had increased to up to 48 percent.

• In 1977, in a hospital in Durban, South Africa, three cases of meningitis and two of septicemia (blood poisoning) were caused by pneumococcal bacteria resistant to both penicillin and chloramphenicol. All three patients with meningitis died. By 1978, this same strain had been isolated from patients in Johannesburg, had acquired additional resistance to erythromycin, tetracycline and cephalosporins, and had caused fourteen deaths. Shortly thereafter, the same resistant strain surfaced in Colorado and Minnesota.

These bacteria from South Africa were even more resistant to penicillin than the earlier examples from Australia and New Guinea, and it was the first report of pneumococci displaying resistance to multiple antibiotics.

"Little by little we are experiencing the erosion of the strongest bulwarks against serious bacterial infections in the modern antibacterial era," wrote Dr. Maxwell Finland of Harvard Medical School in an accompanying editorial to this report in *The New England Journal of Medicine* in 1978. Dr. Finland was one of the world's most respected authorities on infectious disease, and he felt that unless certain steps were taken, we could reach the point of no return.

Two years later, in 1980, Dr. Lewis Thomas, a renowned physician and philosopher, voiced his concern. "I am worried about the future of antibiotics if we do not continue to do research on the appalling problem of antibiotic resistance among our most common pathogens," he wrote. But the warnings of both of these visionaries were largely ignored just as had been the earlier ones from Fleming and Florey.

• In a 1989 survey of several Greek hospitals, the incidence of bacterial antibiotic resistance was extremely high, in some cases up to 100 percent, depending on the type of bacterium and the antibiotic surveyed.

• In Finland, in just two years between 1988 and 1990, the percentage of isolates of streptococci resistant to erythromycin grew rapidly from 4 percent to more than 24 percent.

These are but a few of the hundreds of examples of bacterial antibiotic resistance that have been reported in the past fifty years. Most of them have resulted in treatment failures, and many in deaths. If they are taken as individual, seemingly unrelated occurrences, they appear to be no great cause for alarm.

But they are not unrelated occurrences. They are the result of an insidious process, a bacterial plague that has been an unbroken global chain of events that extends right up until today.

Yet, in 1962, Sir F. Macfarlane Burnet, the Australian immunologist and Nobel laureate whose research paved the way for organ transplantation, wrote that the late twentieth century would be witness to "the virtual elimination of infectious disease as a significant factor in social life." To write about infectious disease, he said, "is almost to write of something that has passed into history." This was echoed seven years later in 1969, when United States Surgeon General William Stewart testified before Congress that it was time to "close the book on infectious diseases." Even as he spoke these words they were being contradicted by scenes being played out in pharmaceutical houses around the world. A crisis that was already in the making in 1969 would explode in the last decade of the twentieth century. But even now, despite the outcries of some of the world's most highly respected scientists, the danger lies buried well beneath the public consciousness.

"The stunning success of the pharmaceutical industry in the United States, Japan, the United Kingdom, France and Germany in creating new antibiotics over the past three decades has caused society and the scientific community to become complacent about the potential of bacterial resistance," said Dr. Harold Neu, an expert in infectious disease and antibiotics at Columbia University School of Medicine. And it is this complacency, believes Dr. Neu, that has put us on the brink of disaster.

Dr. Neu is not alone in his apprehensions. Dr. Richard Krause, senior scientific adviser at the National Institutes of Health and former director of the National Institute of Allergy and Infectious Diseases, said that, based on the increasing number of cases around the world of resistant pneumonia, dysentery, strep, malaria and other diseases, there is only one frightening conclusion that can be drawn: "We have an epidemic of microbial resistance."

But it is Dr. Mitchell Cohen, an infectious disease specialist and epidemiologist at the Centers for Disease Control and Prevention in Atlanta, who sounds the most pessimistic alarm of all, coining a chilling term that may soon become part of our lives. "Unless currently effective antimicrobial agents can be successfully preserved and the transmission of drug-resistant organisms curtailed," he said, "the 'postantimicrobial era' may be rapidly approaching in which infectious disease wards housing untreatable infections will again be seen."

How have we gotten ourselves into such a predicament? This is a complex problem with more heads than Hydra, but at the center of the issue is science, or rather the disregard of science. Therefore, in order to fully appreciate both the problem and what we can do to solve it, we're going to spend the rest of this chapter discussing a little science—how antibiotics work and how bacteria develop resistance to them.

All antibiotics function by interfering with either the structure or the metabolism of a bacterial cell, affecting its ability both to survive and to reproduce. To make an antibiotic therapeutically useful, a basic premise is that the physiologic process to be attacked in the microorganisms should be as different as possible from our own physiology. Obviously it would be a clinical failure to kill or inhibit the growth of bacteria at the cost of a patient's life or well-being.

This is similar to the problem that cancer researchers come up against in trying to develop safe and effective chemotherapeutic agents—those that will attack only cancer cells, while leaving normal tissues untouched. Up till now, however, oncologists have had the more difficult task. Not only have they had fewer anticancer compounds to work with, but it has been more difficult to identify fundamental differences between normal human cells and cancer cells than between human cells and bacteria. Therefore, they have had to rely on drugs that have toxic side effects. Microbial pharmacologists, on the other hand, have had a greater arsenal from which to choose and have been able to be much more selective. From among the thousands of antimicrobial agents known, either derived from natural sources or chemically synthesized in the laboratory, scientists have been able to separate the few hundred that are the most effective and the least toxic. Although some antibiotics still are capable of causing serious side effects, for the most part they are among the safest of all drugs. As we will soon see, this has been both a boon and a bane.

Clinically useful antibiotics can be grouped into several different categories, depending on what part of the bacterial metabolic apparatus they disrupt. One large class prevents bacterial genes from making copies of themselves and from forming the cellular proteins they need to sustain life. Rifampin, one of the antibiotics used to treat tuberculosis, inhibits a specific enzyme that allows bacterial DNA to replicate. A new class of antibiotics, the most popular of which is called ciprofloxacin (trade name Cipro) works in a similar manner. Although our own cells contain a version of the same enzyme, the two types are different enough for the antibiotic not to confuse our cells with bacteria.

Another class of antibiotics, the best-known examples of which are streptomycin, kanamycin, gentamicin and tobramycin, also work in the genetic arena, but in a slightly different way. They interfere with the organization of new bacterial proteins at the main cellular assembly plant called the ribosome. Tetracycline, chloramphenicol and erythromycin and some of the newer relatives are structurally in a slightly different class, but also work by interfering with protein synthesis. Unfortunately, most of the protein-inhibiting antibiotics are not perfect at making the distinction between bacteria and human cells, and it is with this group that we see the most toxic side effects. Streptomycin is rarely used anymore because it can permanently damage hearing. Chloramphenicol is still used around the world to treat typhoid fever, but is almost never used in the United States today because it has a tendency to depress the bone marrow and therefore the formation of new blood cells. And erythromycin causes stomach upset, not so serious a side effect, but still annoying and interfering with the absorption of the antibiotic.

In addition to antibiotics that interfere with the function of genes or the protein synthesis directed by the genes, there are those antibacterial agents that attack bacterial enzymes. The best known of these are the sulfa drugs, chemically synthesized compounds that were first used in the mid-1930s. Sulfa drugs work specifically by inhibiting the formation of the essential chemical folic acid in the bacterial cell without interfering with its formation in human cells.

The best-studied antibiotics belong to the class that interfere with the formation of the bacterial cell wall. These include the penicillins and the cephalosporins. Since human cells don't have a cell wall, these antibiotics are perfectly safe for us (unless we happen to be allergic to them, which is rare).

The penicillins work by inhibiting the enzymes bacteria need to form cross-links in the proteins of their cell wall. Without these crucial cross-links, the bacteria become unstable bags of protoplasm and collapse. Although penicillin doesn't have any affect on adult bacteria, whose cell walls are *already* formed, there is another way they can attack. Most serious infections require that bacteria multiply. Penicillin can deal with that.

RESISTANCE REARS ITS HEAD

Since the historic first successful use of penicillin in March 1941,
a wide variety of penicillin and penicillinlike compounds has been
introduced. The main stimulus for these derivatives and refinements was the clinical observation beginning in the 1950s that
staphylococci, the bacteria that were causing the most serious and
fatal cases of pneumonia and that penicillin was originally most effective against, were rapidly developing resistance to the antibiotic.
Just as Fleming had predicted, staphylococci had now acquired the
enzyme that Abraham and Chain had identified in other bacteria in
1940. What researchers were able to determine was that this enzyme specifically inactivated a portion of the penicillin molecule
known as the beta-lactam ring. By the early 1960s, new penicillins
and the related antibiotic cephalosporin were introduced. These
compounds all worked by stabilizing the beta-lactam ring of the antibiotic, protecting it from attack by the bacteria and preventing
them from developing resistance.

It was assumed that the introduction of these new penicillins
closed a very short book on bacterial resistance. It was comforting
to imagine that through some strange biochemical accident the
staphylococci had managed to develop resistance to penicillin and
that the stabilization of the beta-lactam ring would take care of that
problem once and for all. Virtually everyone in the pharmaceutical
industry congratulated themselves on their ingenuity. Science had
once again triumphed over microorganisms, and this time for good.

The victory, though, proved hollow and extremely short-lived.
The ability of staphylococci to inactivate penicillin enzymatically
wasn't an isolated phenomenon but rather the first example of a
widespread and disturbing trend. Our encounter with bacterial antibiotic resistance hadn't ended. In fact, it was just beginning. Ner-
vous scientists were soon sent back to the laboratory to develop more
antibiotics to circumvent yet another instance of bacterial resistance. And they've been tethered to their workbenches ever since.
Not only did bacteria find a way to become resistant to cephalosporin and the new penicillins, but they began to find ways of becoming resistant to virtually all other antibiotics, old and new. For
the past thirty years we've been engaged in a race with what would

seem the most incongruent of adversaries, unicellular organisms at the far opposite end of the evolutionary spectrum. But in this confrontation, our specialized organs and complicated genetic code put us at a disadvantage. Just as small entrepreneurial companies are often more adept at new product development than the large corporate bureaucracies, so are bacteria quicker to adapt than our more complex systems. Bacteria don't need brains or livers. All they need is the biochemical makeup to become resistant to antibiotics, and for that they are the ultimate gene machines. As Dr. David Perlman, a renowned microbiologist from the University of Wisconsin, has said, "Microorganisms can do anything. Microorganisms are wiser than chemists." Our human hubris has blinded us to the fact that we have never been more than one step ahead of the bacteria and we are in grave danger of losing that slender lead.

This really shouldn't be surprising. Bacteria have had an almost infinite amount of time to become molecularly streamlined, to become far more expert at resisting antibiotics than we are at finding or making them. While antibiotics have been in clinical use for only the past sixty years, bacteria have existed for almost four billion years. And they haven't been lying dormant while the glaciers moved— they've been multiplying and adapting, and doing it, genetically speaking, with blinding speed. A generation of humans is reckoned to be about every twenty years, but bacteria produce progeny every twenty minutes, five hundred thousand times faster than we do. In evolutionary terms, a bacterium that existed in the preantibiotic era of sixty years ago bears the same relationship to one isolated today as does Dryopithecus, the thirty-million-year-old ancestor of humankind, to modern men and women.

After all that time for trial and error, bacteria have come up with essentially three basic biochemical counterattacks against antibiotics. The mechanisms are both elegant and simple. Which one is employed by the bacterium depends on both the type of bacterium and the antibiotic. Often a combination of methods is used on the same antibiotic.

1. Drug inactivation. This is the most common mechanism of resistance to penicillin, ampicillin, amoxicillin (the most widely prescribed drug in the world in 1991) and most of the cephalosporin antibiotics. If you've had any kind of infection in the past five years, especially a urinary or respiratory infection, it's likely your doctor has prescribed a drug in the cephalosporin class. These antibiotics attack the enzyme the bacteria need to stabilize their cell walls, without which they cannot live. As a parry, the bacteria learn to produce another enzyme, whose sole function is to inactivate the antibiotic.

Biochemists have counterattacked with a more advanced class of antibiotics called clavulanates, which prevent the action of this bacterial enzyme. But no one believes that this advantage will prevail. It can't be long before a new generation comes along with yet another enzyme that will render the clavulanates impotent.

Streptomycin and most of the latter-day "mycins," such as tobramycin, gentamicin and kanamycin, are also inactivated by enzymes bacteria produce.

2. Altered target site. Rather than produce an enzyme to neutralize their attacker, bacteria sometimes choose to leave the antibiotic as is and change their own structure instead, usually through mutation. The target bacteria are altered in such a way that the antibiotics can no longer bind to them. The bacteria are, in effect, "hiding" from the antibiotic.

This is another way penicillin and cephalosporin can be rendered ineffective.

3. Metabolic bypass. Rather than destroy the antibiotic or hide from it, in some cases bacteria develop the means to do an end run around the job the antibiotic does. For example, sulfa drugs work by blocking an enzyme bacteria need to make folic acid. But resistant bacteria were able to produce a brand-new enzyme which would allow them to make the crucial folic acid even in the presence of the antibiotic.

Except for a few cases in which scientists haven't yet figured out the mechanisms, almost every one of the reported clinical cases of antibiotic resistance encountered around the world in the past fifty years since the introduction of penicillin—from Japan to Greece to Finland to the United States—has been the result of one or more permutations or refinements by bacteria of these three methods.

As remarkable as all this is as an example of the malleability of an organism, even more remarkable is the way these methods are communicated to other bacteria. Furthermore, bacteria of one species are capable of passing along their biochemical accomplishments to members of other species.

The mechanism bacteria use to thwart the effects of an antibiotic is coded for and directed by a gene. The structure and location of bacterial genes are remarkably similar to those of humans. Just like ours, they are made up of double strands of DNA, and most of them are located on chromosomes. Naturally, bacteria have only a small fraction of the genes we do, but the ones they do possess are responsible for determining all their properties, including antibiotic resistance.

Again similar to what happens to human genes, the bacterial genes on their chromosomes are subject to occasional changes, or mutations. A mutation that imbues a bacterium with an enhanced ability to survive will stick and be passed on from generation to generation.

Mutating is just one thing bacteria are capable of. Bacteria have developed an additional genetic method of becoming resistant that departs completely from anything our own human cells possess. Once in place, this method allows the recipient to quickly spread the wealth far outside its own family. It is this method, in fact, that has been most responsible for the widespread antibiotic resistance we see today and that has finally put us on the brink of disaster.

Although most of the bacterial genes are found on chromosomes, other genes can be found on small circular pieces of DNA outside the chromosome called plasmids. It is here, on the plasmids, that most of the antibiotic-resistance genes are found. One bacterium can carry several types of plasmids; the ones that harbor the genes for antibiotic resistance are called R-plasmids or R-factors. Plasmids can exist autonomously of the parent bacterium; they are almost an organism within an organism. They have a life of their own. They can multiply independently of the bacterium that harbors them and, more important, they can be easily transferred to other bacteria.

One of the ways this transfer takes place is by two bacteria coming into direct contact and exchanging plasmids, the bacterial version of a sexual encounter known as conjugation. Bacteria like to conjugate, but only specialized plasmids can be exchanged by conjugation. If the antibiotic-resistance genes are already on these specialized plasmids, they are smoothly transferred during conjugation. But if they aren't, the bacteria solve the problem by employing another unique molecular tool. Like a genetic flea, tiny pieces of material known as transposons grab on to the R-factors and "hop" from the non-transferable plasmid to the transferable one. This additional step allows virtually all R-factors to be exchanged by conjugation, making it a very efficient way indeed of transferring antibiotic-resistance genes.

Some bacteria, however, that want to transfer their antibiotic-resistance genes simply can't conjugate. Rather than seek counseling, they utilize viral surrogates. These viruses, called bacteriophages, latch onto the R-factors just as do the transposons, but instead of working internally and bringing the genes to a plasmid that can then be transferred by conjugation, the viruses replicate, leave the bacterium and enter another, carrying with them the resistance genes.

By arranging for most resistance genes to be located primarily on plasmids rather than on chromosomes, bacteria have raised the stakes considerably. Antibiotic resistance has changed from the relatively rare clinical occurrences seen in the early days of antibiotic therapy to the explosion of today. Rather than being passed only vertically from mother to daughter cells—as happens if the antibiotic-resistance genes are located on chromosomes—promiscuous bacteria are able to pass R-plasmids to any bacteria they happen to meet up with. Since every one of the more than five billion people in the world carry more bacteria than they do cells, and since bacteria don't need passports to travel, it's not difficult to imagine a scenario whereby bacteria are encountering new and anxious recipients of genetic material all the time. This is why resistance noticed first at one place in the world shows up suddenly and almost simultaneously at a distant corner.

Plasmids and the ease with which they can be transferred among bacteria have been responsible for one other parallel problem, the one that most infectious disease experts believe to be the real challenge of the 1990s: multiple drug resistance. Let's take another look at a few of our earlier examples.

The most significant of them is the almost forty-year-old case of the Japanese woman with dysentery, caused by a *Shigella* bacterium simultaneously resistant to four antibiotics. This phenomenon resulted in more than one epidemic. When it was found that other bacteria—such as normally harmless *E. coli*—which were isolated from the intestinal tracts of infected patients turned out to be resistant to the same four drugs, Tomoichiro Akiba of Tokyo University concluded that resistance had been transferred during conjugation in the patient's digestive tract between the *E. coli* and the shigellae.

Finding multiple-drug-resistant plasmids sitting among normally friendly intestinal bacteria had to mean that they could easily "hitch a ride" to anywhere they chose to go. A few years ago, a study conducted by Dr. Stuart Levy and his colleagues at Tufts University found that almost two-thirds of the stool samples taken randomly from people in the Boston area contained bacteria resistant to at least one antibiotic. This is no longer an unusual finding.

Bacterial resistance to antibiotics is unavoidable. It is a necessary molecular consequence of the use of antibiotics. And no one would suggest that we abandon the use of antibiotics altogether. What we have neglected is finding a balance: a judicious use of antibiotics that would allow the benefits of their use to outweigh the dangers of their misuse. The scale is too heavily tipped toward danger. Physicians have failed to appreciate bacterial physiology and biochemistry. But that is only one part of the problem. The real problem is in the science marketplace.

CHAPTER 2

Hospitals: The Places You Go to Get Sick

It was April 1973. A technologist in the clinical microbiology laboratory of a large Nashville, Tennessee, hospital was logging in the usual array of urine, stool, blood, throat and sputum samples collected from patient wards throughout the hospital, each one coded with a patient identification number. As her next step in this routine, she took sterile cotton swabs and put small amounts of each specimen into petri dishes filled with agar gelatin and nutrients that will support the growth of bacteria. She then placed all the dishes in an incubator with a temperature set at 37° centigrade.

The next morning, the technologist identified the various types of bacteria that had grown. Using a sterile wire loop, she now transferred a bit of each bacterial colony to fresh nutrient-filled petri dishes and around the circumference placed a ring of antibiotic-impregnated discs of filter paper. Everything was incubated overnight again. As the bacteria grew, the antibiotics would diffuse into the agar. If the bacteria were sensitive to the antibiotic, a clear zone of growth inhibition would be visible around the antibiotic-saturated paper the next morning. If the bacteria were resistant, there would be no such zone.

The following day, the technologist reviewed the antibiotic sensitivity results and recorded them on lab slips to be placed on the patient's chart and used as a basis for antibiotic therapy. The technologist is so experienced at her job, she could almost always predict the sensitivity pattern of a particular type of bacterium. But when she checked the petri dish containing bacteria isolated from urine sample #32895, she realized that something was wrong. She had noticed yesterday that the organism that had grown was *Serratia marcescens*, a rather unusual source of urinary infection but one she was now seeing several times a year. What caused her to do a double take wasn't the identification of the *Serratia* itself, but rather the antibiotic sensitivity pattern. There was not one clear zone. This *Serratia* was remarkably resistant. She would have to run the test again, trying other antibiotics. But two days later she had the same results: resistant to everything.

She reported the results to her supervisor, who in turn called the chief of infectious diseases. He decided to monitor the situation closely, but believed it was an isolated medical curiosity, something to be the subject of a future report in the *Journal of Infectious Diseases*. This one patient was in real danger but no further problem was imagined.

Between April and June, things changed. The chief of infectious diseases realized he had underestimated the *Serratia*. Seventeen other patients in the intensive care unit had become infected. Physical control measures—such as strict isolation and increased attention to hand-washing—were intensified. When no more infections were seen in this hospital, it was believed the problem was over, thanks to a simple solution.

But that was *far* from the end of the problem. By October, urinary and respiratory infections with multiply resistant *Serratia* began appearing in a nearby hospital. Since this hospital didn't employ routine surveillance of hospital-acquired infections, the epidemic here went undocumented for an entire year until 128 patients were infected and 5 died. Subsequently, the epidemic spread to two more neighboring hospitals. With physical control measures similar to those instituted earlier, the spread of *Serratia* began to wane, but just as it did, a new wave of urinary and respiratory infections began almost simultaneously in the four hospitals. The culprit this time was not *Serratia*, but another type of bacteria called *Klebsiella*. Tests in the microbiology lab showed that these bacteria were also multiply resistant to antibiotics, and had the same pattern of resistance as the *Serratia*. The final toll by the end of 1974 was more than 400 patients infected by the two organisms with 17 dead.

On the basis of the large outbreak in the second hospital, the Centers for Disease Control in Atlanta was notified, and a group of medical detectives was assembled to begin an investigation. In January 1975, epidemiologists, nurses, microbiologists and infectious disease specialists arrived en masse from Georgia, rendezvoused with physicians from Vanderbilt University Medical Center and began trying to unravel the cause of this major and unusual epidemic.

They were interested primarily in three things: What contributed to the development of the multiply antibiotic-resistant *Serratia*? How was this related to the subsequent epidemic of *Klebsiella*? And how were these resistant strains transmitted to so many patients?

To answer the first question, one part of the team was put in charge of statistical data, looking for common factors among the infected patients that might have promoted growth of the resistant strain. They pored over the charts of the infected patients and tabulated information regarding dates of admission and discharge, diagnosis, length of hospitalization, age, sex, location in the hospital, antibiotic therapy and surgical and medical procedures performed. They also looked at the identification and antibiotic sensitivity records of the hospital microbiology lab dating back several years.

Another group concentrated on the question of transmission. While microbiologists cultured samples from every possible inanimate environmental source of bacteria, from bedpans to bed rails to food carts, staff members were asked to dip their hands into a medium that will encourage the growth of—and thereby reveal the presence of—any *Serratia* or *Klebsiella* on their skin.

The results of the investigation by the CDC eventually confirmed that although *Serratia* had been isolated in the past with varying frequency at each of the four hospitals surveyed, the identification by the technologist in April 1973 marked the first time the highly resistant epidemic strain had been seen. In addition, detailed studies of material sent back to Atlanta revealed that the R-plasmids of the *Serratia* and *Klebsiella* were genetically identical—which meant

that they were somehow linked. Among all the risk factors for a patient developing a clinical infection with *Serratia* or *Klebsiella*, two
soon began to stand out glaringly: previous urinary tract catheterization or surgery and a prior course of broad-spectrum antibiotics.
It all added up in the following way.

The four hospitals in which the epidemic occurred were a short
distance from one another and shared several features. Three of
them were part of an active teaching program at Vanderbilt University Medical Center and shared house staff, medical students, nursing students and other personnel. Subspecialty consultants and
surgeons traveled frequently between these institutions. No source
of inanimate environmental contamination was discovered, but the
hand-washings of personnel were positive for both the antibiotic-
resistant *Serratia* and the *Klebsiella*.

Piecing all of this together, the CDC team developed a scenario.
Urinary catheterization had introduced a nonantibiotic-resistant
Serratia to the original patient. This patient had previously received
a course of broad-spectrum antibiotics and therefore the normal
bacteria in her body already carried genes for antibiotic resistance.
The *Serratia* picked up those genes. Extremely ill with a suppressed
immune system, and with the multiply resistant *Serratia* causing a
urinary infection, this patient was beyond treatment. One or more
of the healthy hospital personnel who came into contact with her
had easily picked up the resistant bacteria on their hands and, although not infected, carried the problem to other patients with suppressed immune systems. Along the way, in one or more patients,
the R-factors containing the antibiotic-resistance genes would be
transferred to a *Klebsiella*, and a new wave of infections and deaths
started to build.

This twenty-year-old epidemic is of more than historical interest. It
provides a prototype for what is happening in our hospitals today. In
many ways, we are even worse off now. When we go into the hospital, we expect to get well, not sick. We expect that conditions there
will be far more antiseptic than in our own homes, not contaminated
with dangerous bacteria. Appallingly, the situation is exactly the opposite.

Hospital-acquired, or nosocomial, infections were not a new phenomenon in 1973. They've been with us for as long as we've had hospitals. But we might expect to have gained some control over them in the one hundred fifty years since Semmelweis, in a nineteenth-century hospital, advocated strict attention to antiseptic technique as a way of preventing birth fever.

As hard as it is to imagine in this age of advanced medical technology, the nosocomial infection rate is at an all-time high and the varieties of infection are becoming ever more serious. Every year, almost two million Americans come down with an infection in a hospital that they didn't have when they entered. More than eighty thousand of them die. This is more than the number of deaths in either the Korean or Vietnam war, more than four times the number killed in auto accidents every year, and more than half as many as have died in the United States from AIDS. It is far from a small matter, yet it's something hospitals would rather you didn't know about. Even in the present climate of keeping the patient informed, see if the next time you or one of your relatives is admitted to a hospital you are told about the very real possibility of acquiring a serious, perhaps even fatal, infection.

Some of the increase in nosocomial infections is unavoidable, a by-product of our own success. In the past few decades, technological advances have changed the practice of medicine. In our story of the *Serratia* and *Klebsiella* epidemic, a urinary catheter was the conduit for the bacteria to enter the body and an immunosuppressed patient provided a fertile ground for growth. Hospitals in the nineties use more catheters than ever, and many different kinds. And we also are treating more immunosuppressed people than ever: patients with AIDS, multiple-trauma victims, elderly patients.

But by far the main reason we are seeing so many serious nosocomial infections is the nearly exponential increase in the use of antibiotics over the past few decades. In 1962 hospitals in the United States purchased $94 million worth of antibiotics; in 1971 the corresponding figure was $218 million; by 1991 the number had exploded tenfold to $3 billion; and by 1997 it is projected that annual sales of antibiotics to hospitals will top $8 billion! Most of the antibiotics used today are broad-spectrum antibiotics, effective against many different types of bacteria. The broader the spectrum of the antibiotics, the more we depend on them. Paradoxically, the more effective antibiotics become at wiping out a wide range of bacteria, the better than ever they become at supporting the growth of resistant strains.

There is a scientific principle called *selection pressure* that we now have to understand. But first we must point out that the acquisition of an antibiotic-resistance gene is not by itself sufficient to make bacteria dangerous. The resistance gene is necessary—but there is more to the story.

Let's explore further some of the details of the 1973 Nashville epidemic. The patient from whom the first multiply resistant *Serratia* was isolated had been given a previous course of broad-spectrum antibiotics. Prior to the administration of those antibiotics, among the billions of bacteria that populated her body (we all normally carry billions of bacteria), there were only a few that carried multiple-antibiotic-resistance genes, having come to reside there by natural mutation. These antibiotic-resistant bacteria were not *Serratia*. They were an ordinary, non-disease-causing variety, and they weren't having an easy time surviving. They had to compete for very limited nutrients with antibiotic-*sensitive* bacteria, which outnumbered the resistant ones at least a million to one and which were formidable competitors. The antibiotic-resistant bacteria had no advantage. But this changed when broad-spectrum antibiotics were administered. Now the playing field was no longer level. The antibiotics became the allies of the *resistant* bacteria, killing off the sensitive ones and clearing a path for the nutrients. Generation after generation multiplied and thrived. (In the world of bacteria, a new generation comes along every twenty minutes.) The advantage the antibiotics were able to confer on the resistant bacteria is called *selection pressure*.

Still, in order for a dangerous infection to develop, these resistant genes had to first be transferred from the "ordinary variety" to a more virulent organism, virulent enough to cause disease. Enter the *Serratia* via the urinary catheter. In the past *Serratia* had been known as tame and ubiquitous hospital residents. But that was before they met up with the "ordinary" bacteria carrying the resistant genes. Now, taking the resistant genes, they became devils. And as more patients with suppressed immune systems began to populate the hospitals, *Serratia*—now devils—could join the group of organisms causing opportunistic infections. These bacterial villains prey on cancer patients, AIDS patients, the debilitated elderly and anyone else who can't fight back.

Being pathogens, they would have done this even if they *hadn't* had the opportunity to acquire the antibiotic-resistance genes. But in their former molecular state the *Serratia* were still sensitive to many antibiotics, so the infections they caused would have been relatively easy to treat. Now, newly armed, they were able to cause a urinary infection that was impossible to treat. It was the recognition of what this could mean that had sent a wave of apprehension through the Nashville hospital microbiology laboratory. And the fear heightened when it was later realized that in their travels the *Serratia* had conjugated with and shared their genes for multiple antibiotic resistance with *Klebsiella*, which had a greater propensity to populate the respiratory tract and cause pneumonias. They were thus even more dangerous than the *Serratia*.

Once the resistant *Serratia* multiplied in this patient in large numbers, they had an easy time hitching a ride on the hands and in the nasal passages of the hospital workers. Thus a chain reaction of transmission to vulnerable patients in other hospitals—the epidemic—began.

Here we've seen just one example of what widespread damage bacteria can do when they can't be stopped by any antibiotic. Ever since the first recognition of R-plasmids and multiple antibiotic resistance in 1955, the identification of these invulnerable microorganisms has been increasing. And it's not just because we've become better at detecting them. Primarily because of the dramatic increase in antibiotic use, especially broad-spectrum antibiotics, the actual number of resistant bacteria in hospital infections is accelerating at an alarming rate. As of today, not every hospital-acquired infection is caused by bacteria resistant to all or almost all available antibiotics, but we are getting closer and closer to that frightening reality every year.

One's worries have to intensify when resistant strains become genetically stronger. When such a gene first comes to reside on a plasmid, it finds itself not in the most stable location. If the gene doesn't improve its position, it is likely at some point to be displaced. It would then lose its easy transferability to other bacteria. But through selection pressure the gene can be moved to a strategically better neighborhood. Eventually, after enough administrations of antibiotic to enough people, the antibiotic-resistance gene comes to occupy the best house on the plasmid block. There's no dislodging it once that happens.

Besides stabilizing already resistant strains, selection pressure causes the emergence of new and different resistant bacteria. This has been reflected in the changing types of bacteria that have predominated in hospital infections over the past four decades. Every few years another resistant strain steps forward and with each changing of the guard, the resistance vise tightens its grip on us, propelling us closer and closer to where most infections are untreatable.

Before the introduction of antibiotics, staphylococci were responsible for most hospital infections, primarily pneumonias. Throughout most of the 1940s these were well controlled by the vigorous use of penicillin. During that period, while patients were being cured, selection pressure was also taking place behind the scenes, and the few penicillin-resistant staph that had existed prepenicillin began to take over. By the 1950s these new penicillin-resistant strains of staph emerged with a vengeance and a dramatic resurgence of infections once again plagued hospitals.

Then in the early 1960s, methicillin and cephalosporin were introduced, which eventually subdued the penicillin-resistant staph. This time the staph proved not as resilient; they didn't bounce back as easily as they had against the original penicillin. The staph were sent back to their lairs to lick their wounds and regroup.

But that was far from the end of nosocomial infections. With staph temporarily out of the picture, other players called gram-negative bacteria began to take over as the main hospital pathogens. One way bacteria can be quickly categorized under the microscope is according to whether or not they absorb a stain, called the Gram stain. Staph do and are gram-positive; those that don't are gram-negative.

Serratia and *Klebsiella* are gram-negative bacteria and it was in the 1970s that they, along with several other gram-negative bacteria, began to make their presence felt. These infections were even more deadly than the staph infections, killing up to 30 percent of those stricken. In the 1970s a powerful new antibiotic called gentamicin was introduced, and it, along with some other closely related drugs, was able to subdue many gram-negative infections. But not all of them. The *Serratia-Klebsiella*-resistant-to-everything incident occurred nevertheless.

As many of the gram-negative bacteria were pushed out the revolving door in the 1980s, the staph reentered, this time with more muscle than ever before: they were now resistant to methicillin. MRSA (methicillin-resistant *Staphylococcus aureus*) became the most dreaded abbreviation ever to haunt microbiologists and infectious disease specialists. With all the selection pressure from different antibiotics that the staph had been exposed to over the decades, they had been able to augment their natural resistance to many antibiotics with acquired genes. These organisms began to cause scores of infections, including pneumonias, serious wound infections in surgical patients, septicemia (blood poisoning) in burn patients (a group especially susceptible to these bacteria), and the elderly in long-term care facilities.

Physicians were caught off guard. There were no effective antibiotics to treat these patients. Once again, the pharmaceutical industry showed remarkable ingenuity and developed new antibiotics, but the optimism was short-lived. Ciprofloxacin (Cipro), introduced in 1987, was hailed as a savior, but the methicillin-resistant staph quickly developed resistance. Therefore, by the late 1980s, the options for treatment of these bacteria had narrowed considerably; physicians were down to just one antibiotic, and it was one they didn't want to use.

The name of this antibiotic was vancomycin. Vancomycin was not new. It had been discovered in 1956 but rarely administered. Specialists always kept it in the back of the antibiotic closet—and their minds. Not only was it toxic, but its mechanism of action against certain bacteria, especially staph, had led to the widespread belief that it might really be the final *reinforcement* against resistant bacteria. If vancomycin had to be used, just as all other antibiotics, it too would eventually select for resistant strains, and then where would we be? But the MRSA were forcing physicians' hands. They had no choice but to roll out the heavy artillery.

And to make matters even worse, in the early 1980s the methicillin-resistant staph began to bring along some cousins called enterococci against which vancomycin would also have to be used, increasing the chances for vancomycin resistance.

As vancomycin use escalated through the 1980s, the inevitable finally happened. In 1988 and 1989 there were reports from institutions around the world of a rash of infections resistant to vancomycin, the villains being the very same cousins of the methicillin-resistant staph. Our hospitals were now plagued by organisms which, like the *Serratia* and *Klebsiella* in Nashville twenty years earlier, were resistant to all antibiotics. More aggressive, they were a threat to robust patients as well as weakened ones. Theoretically everyone in the hospital was a target.

Today, along with *Serratia* and other gram-negative bacteria, methicillin-resistant staph and its cousins are among the most common causes of nosocomial infections. The very real worry among infectious disease specialists is that the methicillin-resistant staph will soon acquire the vancomycin resistance gene from its cousins and the armory of possible treatments will be totally depleted. Physicians in the know are privately wringing their hands. For the first time in more than fifty years, they are faced with the antibiotic cupboard being completely bare.

It's bad enough that such things are happening in our hospitals. But are we any safer outside of them? Pathologists use hospital microbiology laboratories to grow and isolate bacteria, and to check them for antibiotic sensitivity. At the same time, however, bacteria have commandeered the entire hospital as their own personal research and development laboratory. Since antibiotic use is greatest—and therefore selection pressure is greatest—in the hospital, and since patients are most susceptible, it has become the perfect proving ground for bacteria to hone old genes and try out new ones. And once they have been tested under fire, they are ready to venture out into the community and try their hand on the rest of us.

The worst of the drug-resistant infections are those transmitted by the fecal-oral route such as shigellosis, foodborne illnesses such as salmonellosis, sexually transmitted diseases such as gonorrhea and *Chlamydia*, and certain respiratory infections, especially pneumonia.

In the past few years, shigellosis has become a serious problem affecting Native American populations, children in day care and homosexual men. Most of these cases are accompanied by mild diarrhea and fever and do not require antibiotic treatment, but drugs are often given anyway. And it has been known for decades that multiple drug resistance in *Shigella* emerges and spreads rapidly (remember that the first case of multiple drug resistance and R-plasmids ever discovered in the 1950s was in a case of *Shigella* and that several serious epidemics followed), yet physicians have failed to appreciate the lesson and use restraint in prescribing antibiotics.

A warning was issued as early as 1973 by Dr. J. E. M. Whitehead in an article in the *British Medical Journal*.

Indiscriminate prescribing of antibiotics, whether inside or outside hospitals, adds needlessly to the mounting pressures for selection of resistant organisms. It may seem an overstatement to describe it as an act of environmental pollution, but when the full and ultimate consequences of this manner of use are grasped, it is less of an exaggeration than might at first appear. What makes for rational chemotherapy is the prescribing of antibacterial drugs only where there are valid clinical indications and when attention is paid to the current resistance patterns of the probable pathogens.

In 1978, Dr. Calvin Kunin, chief of infectious disease at Ohio State University and currently chairman of the Infectious Disease Society of America's committee on antibiotics, added to Dr. Whitehead's warning when he said "Antibiotic usage conjures up an image of fallout akin to that from a leaking nuclear reactor."

When Dr. Whitehead wrote his condemnation the situation in our hospitals was already appalling. But despite the establishment in the

United States shortly thereafter of a National Task Force on the Clinical Use of Antibiotics (under Dr. Kunin's guidance), things did not improve.

Today, approximately 35 percent of patients in hospitals receive at least one antibiotic during their stay. And almost half the patients in the surgical and pediatric wards receive them routinely. Up to two-thirds of these patients show no evidence of infection. This doesn't mean that all of them are being given antibiotics inappropriately. But the prophylactic administration of antibiotics—the prescribing of an antibiotic to prevent an infection rather than to treat it—does account for 50 percent of use.

Moreover, about 35 percent of the time the wrong drug is prescribed in treating presumed infections. And when the wrong drug is used, more often than not it is a broad-spectrum antibiotic, one that is most efficient in eliminating sensitive bacteria and fostering the growth of resistant strains.

The prophylactic use of antibiotics in hospitals is a subject of much discussion these days. For a long time, infectious disease specialists and surgeons have been at war over the proper prophylactic use of antibiotics, with patients the victims and antibiotic-resistant bacterial strains the beneficiaries. Dr. Kunin of Ohio State has written that there is probably no issue in antimicrobial therapy that is more emotionally charged than the prophylactic use of antibiotics.

The majority of prophylactic antibiotics are given to surgical patients. Antimicrobial prophylaxis clearly has an important place in surgery. Postoperative wound infections affect at least 920,000 of the 23 million patients who undergo surgery each year in the United States. The rates of infection vary according to the procedure: from less than 3 infections per 100 cases for "clean procedures" (those in which there is no violation of aseptic technique during the operation and the digestive, respiratory and urinary systems are not entered) to up to 9 infections per 100 cases for both grossly contaminated procedures and "dirty cases" (those in which the digestive, respiratory and urinary systems are entered). For some operations, such as gallbladder removal via nonlaparoscopic surgery, the rate may be increased fivefold. The fact that most surgical patients receive antibiotics doesn't by itself constitute inappropriate use at all. The problem is in the choice of the antibiotics and the length of time they are given.

Elegant studies more than thirty years ago demonstrated that the timing of the prophylaxis is critical. To be effective in preventing postoperative infection, the antibiotic must be given before the procedure—prophylaxis is completely ineffective if given only postoperatively—and only a very short course is required. Until 1992, a short course meant forty-eight hours before the operation, but a study in *The New England Journal of Medicine* from the University of Utah showed that prophylactic antibiotics are most effective if given during the two-hour period just before the surgical incision. In this study, not only was there no added benefit from giving antibiotics at any other time but the rates of infection were shown to be greater if antibiotics were initiated either more than two hours preoperatively or at any time postoperatively.

Studies have also shown that, in order to be most effective, the choice of antibiotic must be tailored to the operation. The known common invaders of the female genital tract are different from those expected in orthopedic or cardiovascular surgery, and hence the antibiotics used for prophylaxis should be chosen accordingly. And the dose for prophylaxis need not be large. It must simply produce blood levels that will inhibit the common invading organisms. One of the most complete studies in support of this conclusion was performed in the division of infectious disease at the University of Wisconsin Medical Center in 1978 and these results still hold today. The appropriateness of the therapy was judged according to very rigid and specific criteria that had been set up earlier by a national group headed by Dr. Kunin. In the cases where prophylaxis was listed as the reason for giving antibiotics, it was judged inappropriate in almost half the cases, usually because the course of antibiotics was unduly prolonged.

Even though it is well documented that the short course is the right approach, clinical surveys have indicated that physicians pay almost no attention to this. Patients entering the hospital for surgery of any kind are invariably given an antibiotic practically the moment they arrive on the surgical floor. And this is usually continued until the day they are discharged (and sometimes even afterward), no matter how long their hospital stay.

Although antibiotics are rarely dispensed by office-based physicians for prophylactic reasons, other rationales are found for profligate prescribing. In 1991, physicians in the United States wrote almost 240 million prescriptions for antibiotics, one for every person in the country. Naturally some of these were justified and appropriate. But if we break down the figures a little, we can see that, analogous to what happens in our hospitals, not only were many antibiotics dispensed unnecessarily, but the wrong ones were used.

Perhaps the worst indictment of all is that more than 900,000 antibiotic prescriptions were written when the diagnosis was a common cold. You don't need a medical degree to know that antibiotics are completely ineffective against viral infections such as colds, and there is little evidence to justify giving an antibiotic to prevent a secondary infection. Something is at work here besides sound medical judgment. And this statistic is drawn only from those physicians honest enough to admit they were prescribing an antibiotic for a cold. Others, perhaps more aware that prescriptions are audited nationally, used vague and creative diagnoses such as "acute respiratory infection, unspecified" (more than 1.5 million prescriptions), "allergic rhinitis, unspecified" (700,000 prescriptions) and "chronic rhinitis" (600,000). If we assume that most of these are synonyms for colds, then there were almost four million prescriptions written in 1991 for the common cold, and it's likely that practically all were unnecessary.

And the kinds of antibiotics prescribed by practicing physicians reflect the same trend seen everywhere in medicine: the increased use of broad-spectrum drugs, to the point where it's almost a curiosity when a narrow-spectrum antibiotic is used. Of the 240 million antibiotic prescriptions, more than 170 million, 71 percent, were in the broad-spectrum category. The majority of these were amoxicillin and cephalosporins.

Antibiotics have become what Dr. Kunin has called "drugs of fear." Physicians have come to believe that broad-spectrum antibiotics are effective against almost any infection. They fear that if they don't treat, they may very well be overlooking an infection that is not yet visible or producing symptoms. Since many physicians also fear legal action, administering antibiotics is frequently seen as the appropriate way to practice defensive medicine. But given their role in the advent of new and life-threatening resistant bacteria, "drugs of fear" could soon take on a whole new meaning.

CHAPTER 3

Apocalypse Soon?

Tommy was a beautiful one-year-old boy who lived with his mother, sister and brother in a poor section of Houston. Their two-room apartment was a tight fit for the family, even though it was less crowded now than it had been before Tommy's father disappeared a month after his son's birth. Tommy's mother would have kept Tommy in the same room with her anyway to protect the sleep of his siblings, but she was the more anxious to have him near because he'd been sick for the past three months. Late one night the sounds of explosive coughing and noisy wheezing summoned her to her baby's bed. When she saw that his lips were blue, she bundled him up and rushed him to the nearest hospital emergency room.

The young mother had already journeyed repeatedly to every out-patient clinic and emergency room in search of an explanation for Tommy's breathing problem. Most of the doctors provided children's aspirin, advice to drink plenty of fluids and reassuring admonitions to be patient. One suspected some type of pneumonia and prescribed an antibiotic that controls many community-acquired lung pathogens. But even she didn't order a chest x-ray, because she doubted that the stingy Medicaid program in Texas would pay for the procedure. Nor did anyone perform a tuberculin skin test, which should have been standard for any patient having an acute respiratory problem, especially if he was impoverished. It would have been positive.

On this rainy night, Tommy's severe symptoms finally forced the doctors to perform a thorough diagnostic workup which pointed strongly to tuberculosis. But it was too late. The infection had already turned to an aggressive disease that easily marched throughout the infant's body. Twenty hours after admission to the hospital, Tommy died with widespread, multidrug-resistant tuberculosis.

In the sad aftermath of Tommy's death, the Houston Department of Health conducted an investigation. They learned that unknown to Tommy's mother, his father had been told he had tuberculosis three weeks before the birth. He began taking isoniazid and rifampin, two powerful antituberculosis antibiotics, but left the pills in the apartment when he walked out. Before deserting, he had transmitted *Mycobacterium tuberculosis* to the newborn.

Tommy's story is not pretty, but it can teach us much. Tuberculosis illuminates so clearly how both intellectual and moral failures have combined to create our crisis of bacterial resistance. It is also, among all the diseases that have developed antibiotic resistance, the first that is both deadly and has the potential to spread explosively to a very large part of the U.S. population.

Tuberculosis has been familiar to humankind since before the time of Hippocrates. Reliable accounts say this single disease caused at least 20 percent of the deaths in London in 1651 and up to a third of all deaths in Paris in the early nineteenth century. As recently as the beginning of this century, *Mycobacterium tuberculosis* accounted for 15 percent of all adult deaths in the United States.

After thousands of years, the tide turned against this killer in 1882. The founding of the first tuberculosis sanatorium in Saranac Lake, New York, in that year began a century-long decline in cases. Sanatoriums didn't possess effective drugs, and owed their impact mainly to the emphasis they placed on good ventilation and outdoor activities. The explanation lies in the way the tuberculosis pathogen makes its way from person to person.

People who contract tuberculosis do so by inhaling *Mycobacterium tuberculosis* that someone with the disease has coughed or sneezed into the air. Although tuberculosis disseminates in the same way as a cold or the flu, it isn't nearly as contagious. You're not likely ever to get it outdoors or from any stranger with whom you sit through a movie or concert. Careful experimental observations have shown that people generally need to be exposed to a concentrated source of bacteria for a considerable length of time in a crowded, poorly ventilated area—such as Tommy's apartment—in order to become infected. When patients in sanatoriums coughed, by contrast, the bacteria they launched tended to dissipate harmlessly into the air and die when exposed to the ultraviolet spectrum of sunlight. Hence the patients didn't keep fueling their disease by reinhaling their own or each other's microbes. In addition, of course, they were less likely to transmit their infection to family and friends they left behind when they entered the institution.

In the early 1950s, the decline of tuberculosis accelerated sharply as new antibiotics rendered it a curable disease. Most treatment schedules involve six months of taking daily doses of isoniazid and rifampin, and sometimes pyrazinamide. The fact that this is commonly referred to as a "short course" points up how difficult tuberculosis bacteria are to eradicate. Until recently, 90 percent of the patients who took all their pills were rewarded with a cure.

These successful results lulled everyone into letting their guard down. The sanatoriums closed or were converted to nursing homes or even resorts. Government-sponsored research on tuberculosis dried up. The most promising medical students set their sights on cardiology and neurology, where the action was hot. Long before Surgeon General Stewart's ill-advised 1969 statement claiming victory over infectious diseases, a consensus prevailed that the United States had licked tuberculosis as a serious public health problem.

Most physicians from developed countries, myself included, were convinced. As a pathologist I have performed close to one thousand autopsies, many of them in county and university hospital settings that serve the indigent populations who are most susceptible to tuberculosis. To this day the only direct contacts I've had with the erstwhile scourge were on microscopic slides from the departmental archives. I recall one time when a neighboring hospital announced that it had a case, and several of us hurried across town to see it firsthand, almost as if we were on some archaeological dig in search of this medical relic from the nineteenth century.

Nevertheless, the medical community's complacency was completely inappropriate, and thousands of patients are paying for it today. To understand what is happening, we need first to look at how tuberculosis operates. For most communicable illnesses we have to distinguish between infection and disease. Infection simply means that an organism has entered our body. Our immune defenses may squash an infection, or it may remain dormant. Disease occurs when an infection becomes aggressive, invading and destroying tissues and causing symptoms. This difference is especially important when considering tuberculosis.

Once infected with *Mycobacterium tuberculosis,* people may develop disease by either of two basic patterns. The first is rare, occurring in very young children and immunocompromised adults. In the absence of a strong immune response, the bacteria pass from the lungs right into the bloodstream, whence they give rise to disseminated disease and lethal tuberculous meningitis.

In the great majority of people, the route from infection to disease is more tenuous. White blood cells called macrophages, which are the first-line sentinels of the immune system, attack the inhaled bacteria as they land in the lungs. The macrophages ingest some of the invaders and besiege the rest within small, localized nodules called tubercles. (The name *tuberculosis* derives from these tiny scablike formations in the lungs, which were first discovered by Franciscus Sylvius in 1679.) During the two to six weeks after the initial infection, the body manufactures T-cells that are specifically adapted to seek out and destroy *Mycobacterium tuberculosis.* These and other specialized components of the immune system infiltrate into the tubercle, kill off most but not all of the remaining sequestered bacteria, and reinforce—calcify—the walls of the tubercle.

Throughout this entire struggle, as a rule, the infected person never notices any symptoms. In most cases, the only way to know that infection has occurred is to scratch a solution of proteins derived from *Mycobacterium tuberculosis* into the patient's skin. A doctor or nurse can then observe the formation of a rash as the programmed T-cells rush to the site. Some people do not develop a rash when challenged with the tuberculin skin test, but x-rays betray the infection by showing the healed, calcified tubercles.

So far, the infected individual is still healthy, and in fact 90 percent will remain so throughout their lives. Nevertheless, some bacteria still survive within the calcified tubercle. Should the tubercle wall crumble, they will break out and spread through the lymph channels or bloodstream. This is what happens to one infected person in ten. Most often, the freed bacteria lodge in the top of the lung, lymph nodes, brain, bones, kidneys, adrenal glands, or skin. The immune system rallies again, of course, but cannot be as successful against the bacteria now that they are established as it was when they were newly arrived in the lung. The host becomes sick with fever, fatigue and wasting—the vivid sapping of life force that gave the disease one of its most telling nicknames, "consumption"—along with chest pain, hoarseness and eventually a bloody cough. When tuberculosis reaches this stage, it is fatal more than 50 percent of the time. Yet even those patients who die can transmit the infection to, quite commonly, ten or more people if the conditions are right.

Because of this complex natural history, Americans retained a high degree of vulnerability to tuberculosis even when the disease fell to its lowest ebb in the 1970s. A large number of people who had never experienced tubercular symptoms harbored bacteria from previous infections and were at risk of becoming sick if their natural resistance declined.

Enter HIV infection and AIDS. Taking advantage of these patients' immunosuppressed status, tuberculosis can be a jackal that ravenously devours their tissues in incredibly short periods of time. Patients with AIDS who develop tuberculosis often die in one to four months. An insidious feature of advanced HIV is that it makes tuberculosis infection difficult to diagnose. The virus decimates the T-cells whose reaction is what makes a tuberculin skin test positive. In a curious reversal, a positive tuberculin test may be one of the earliest visible clues to the diagnosis of HIV in patients who still have an appreciable number of T-cells.

More than one million HIV-positive people in the United States alone have provided a fertile feeding ground for the tuberculosis bacterium. Add to these at least another million people who are immunosuppressed because of some combination of intravenous drug abuse, malnutrition and chronic infections, and it's plain to see how tuberculosis made its comeback.

An even larger factor in the new tuberculosis epidemic is old-fashioned neglect. Having vanquished the disease conceptually with their antibiotics, the medical establishment developed the illusion that it had eradicated it in fact. Content to live in obscurity, tuberculosis persisted in the poorest sections of New York City, Miami, Houston and Atlanta. While the rest of the country forgot about the disease, these and other big American urban centers reported a steady stream of cases throughout the 1960s, 1970s and 1980s. In 1970, for example, residents of Harlem sustained almost twenty times as much active tuberculosis as the national average, and five times more than the rest of New York City.

In 1985, the combination of a growing population of immunosuppressed individuals and spillover from unrecognized reservoirs of disease combined to bring our national decline in tuberculosis to a screeching halt. Cases began to rise again—sharply. Between 1985 and 1991, the increase was almost 20 percent nationwide, with almost 27,000 cases reported in 1991. Besides causing tremendous pain and suffering, they will add billions of dollars to a health care system already strained to its fiscal limit. The American Lung Association now somberly predicts that unless we launch a major concerted effort, within a decade we will be seeing in excess of 50,000 new cases of tuberculosis each year.

This resurgence is not limited to the United States; in fact, it is even more marked in some other countries. In the past five years, reported cases of tuberculosis have shot up 33 percent in Switzerland, 30 percent in Denmark and 28 percent in Italy.

Nestled among these grim statistics is the bleak fact that the group experiencing the fastest rise is children like Tommy. Between 1985 and 1990, the largest jump in tuberculosis rates was in children ages five to fourteen years. For children less than five years old, the incidence increased a dramatic 39 percent between 1989 and 1992. Outbreaks of tuberculosis have been occurring in day care centers and schools. In a recent outbreak in a St. Louis elementary school, thirty-eight children developed pulmonary tuberculosis. Almost half of the students who didn't become ill were found to be infected.

Except for a few voices in the wilderness, the return of tuberculosis surprised almost all health authorities, from government officials to physicians to researchers. Beginning in 1987, after the Centers for Disease Control audits identified the increased number of cases and an alarming incidence of resistance to the standard antituberculosis drugs, a flurry of activity commenced in an attempt to head off a growing threat.

Most of us didn't become aware that anything untoward was going on until we read newspaper stories in late 1991. Shortly thereafter, in April 1992, a two-day public hearing was held in Washington. Called "Tuberculosis: Return of an Epidemic," it was chaired by the late New York Congressman Ted Weiss. Medical experts working in the tuberculosis trenches from hospitals in New York, Miami and Houston testified, decrying the blindness of governmental policies and decades of lack of basic support for research into this problem. One after another, they stressed the absolute necessity of reversing the trend immediately. The desperation in their voices and words was palpable. Although William Roper, the director of the Centers for Disease Control, and Anthony Fauci, the director of the National Institute for Allergy and Infectious Disease, responded by outlining specific plans that were already implemented and others that were promised soon, the scientists still seemed skeptical.

The support systems had been allowed to deteriorate to the point that in 1992 our national tuberculosis policy structure was a gutted edifice. Despite having physicians as concerned and competent as Roper and Fauci on the right side of the issue, with government bureaucracy in charge it is difficult to be optimistic about how quickly results can be expected.

The revival of tuberculosis has doctors and nurses stepping more gingerly around patients—and inhaling more tentatively—than ever before. Knowledgeable caregivers realize they're much more likely to pick up *Mycobacterium tuberculosis* from a patient who has consumption than they are to contract human immunodeficiency virus from one with AIDS. Furthermore, if they should become sick from a strain of bacteria that is drug-resistant, tuberculosis may be the more rapidly fatal of the two diseases.

The mortality rate for tuberculosis that resists two or more antibiotics is between 40 and 60 percent, just about the same as prevailed before antibiotics. Telling patients today that they have contracted multidrug-resistant tuberculosis is equivalent to telling patients fifty years ago that they had developed pneumonia or meningitis. The chances of surviving are about the same.

Bacterial resistance is the new and chilling feature in the current tuberculosis epidemic. A recent Greater New York Hospital Association survey of hospitalized tuberculosis patients indicated that 46 percent of tuberculosis bacteria isolated resisted at least one, and more often two or more, of the drugs doctors had always relied on. Although New York City leads the United States in drug-resistant cases, the problem exists nationwide. Treatment failures have been reported in at least thirty-six states, the District of Columbia, and Puerto Rico.

To appreciate how tuberculosis becomes resistant, we have to introduce a variant of the selection pressure principle. Just as administering antibiotics when they aren't needed can foster the development of resistant strains by eliminating their competition, so can what takes place at the other end of the spectrum—that is, not taking antibiotics when they are required or not taking them for as long as they are required. Here we cannot indict the medical profession for the inappropriate use of antibiotics; it is Tommy's father and others on the receiving end who are using them wrongly. The microbial scenario differs somewhat, but the results are the same.

Remember that every population of organisms includes a small number of strains that are resistant to some antibiotic. If an infected person takes that particular antibiotic, it will knock out all the organisms except the perhaps one in a thousand that is resistant. This genetically lucky bacterium evades the pharmaceutical holocaust that takes its relatives, but two factors keep it from immediately capitalizing on the lack of competition. The presence of the antibiotic in the environment hems it in, and it still has to contend with the immune system. In general, as long as the patient keeps taking the drug, her white blood cells will mop up the few isolated nonsusceptible microbes. She'll be cured.

A large number of patients, however, don't stay the course with their antibiotic therapy. Most start off highly motivated by distressing symptoms—fever, night sweats, a relentless, hammering cough and generalized weakness. The symptoms wane after only a couple weeks of therapy, however, and the patient naturally begins to feel less urgency about taking every pill. Like Tommy's father, many simply stop taking their medication at this stage, even though they still have over five months to go to truly eradicate the infection. In most surveys of large cities, less than 50 percent of patients on antibiotics for tuberculosis complete their prescribed course of medication.

A partial course of prescribed antibiotics, called a subtherapeutic dose, creates a perfect situation for the selection of antibiotic-resistant bacteria. When the patient abandons treatment, *Mycobacterium tuberculosis* reasserts itself. Resistant strains now predominate, and with neither competition nor antibiotics to deter them, they take over the store. The patient falls ill again, but this time the drugs don't work.

Immunosuppression, like poor compliance, fosters resistant strains. Children and people with HIV lack the white cells needed to eliminate the bacteria the antibiotic misses.

Resistant tuberculosis strains have grown strong enough to break out of the relapsed and weakened populations that first incubated them. They now cause many first-time infections in people with normal immunity. A study of 466 patients in New York City revealed that resistant bacteria were responsible for over 70 percent of initial infections. Thomas Frieden, the director of New York City's Bureau of Tuberculosis Control, commented: "Most people with multidrug-resistant tuberculosis got it from bad luck, not because they were bad at taking their medicines."

The process of amassing drug-resistant tuberculosis strains and transmitting them to the healthy is transpiring robustly in prisons. "The surge in incarceration rates and long sentences due to stricter drug laws has filled prisons with inmates who are infected with tuberculosis and HIV," says John Rabba, former director of Cermak Health Services, the health care provider for Chicago's Cook County jail. "By cramming more people who are immunocompromised into tremendously overcrowded and poorly ventilated facilities, we have set the table for a terrible dinner of tuberculosis to serve the public."

Nearly all prisoners eventually return to their communities. Correction officers go home every day to their families. Both can unknowingly be carrying lethal resistant tuberculosis bacteria. A tuberculosis flash fire broke out in an Arkansas state prison and spread to the community when a released inmate infected his wife and two children, one of whom died of tuberculous meningitis. In 1990, a New York City news reporter discovered she had been infected while working on a story on the outbreak of multidrug-resistant tuberculosis at the jail on Rikers Island. This complex has one of the highest tuberculosis case rates in the nation.

The real nightmare, however, will visit us if drug-resistant strains escape our borders into the developing nations. Had the American medical community occasionally doffed our industrialized-nation blinders and looked at the rest of the world, we could never have made the mistake of turning our backs on this disease. The stark reality is that as a global problem, tuberculosis has never retreated an inch. Infectious illnesses remain the number one global cause of death, and tuberculosis heads the list. To those of us insulated from sub-Saharan Africa, India, Latin America and the rest of the developing world, the statistics can be staggering. Each year worldwide there are an estimated ten million new cases of tuberculosis and three million deaths from the disease. Tuberculosis chalks up almost 7 percent of all deaths in the developing world, and almost 20 percent of deaths in adults aged fifteen to fifty-nine. All told, approximately one-third of the world's population, more than one and a half billion people, harbors *Mycobacterium tuberculosis*. Should drug-resistant strains come to prevail in this enormous reservoir, tuberculosis has the potential to sow death on a truly millennial scale.

Other resistant bacterial diseases have put us at the edge of danger, but tuberculosis has put us over the edge. In addition to its direct menace, it has given us a frightening vision of how other plagues may arise if we don't begin to act immediately. Although tuberculosis is a unique disease with features unlike virtually any other infection, it is a barometer. If we fail to stem the tide here, there is little reason to be optimistic about controlling other infectious epidemics looming on our horizon.

To doctors trained in my generation, whose eyes have been on the unfolding world of gene therapy and computerized imaging, it's hard to shake the sense of a strange anachronism when talking of tuberculosis. Yet there it stands as a testament to our shortsightedness and provincial thinking.

The problem is not really with tuberculosis so much as with the devilish way in which antibiotics have turned on us and in a real sense become the enemy. One day soon, biomedical research will find a new way to deal with resistant strains of tuberculosis. As an important and widely hailed first step, in August 1992, in the British journal *Nature,* researchers from Hammersmith Hospital in London and at the Institut Pasteur in Paris reported they had identified at the molecular level exactly how *Mycobacterium tuberculosis* becomes resistant to isoniazid. And in 1993, microbiologists from Albert Einstein Medical College in New York and the University of Pittsburgh devised an ingenious test to detect resistant strains of tuberculosis bacteria in the laboratory within just a few days after culturing a sputum sample, in contrast to the two to three months required by standard tests. The assay involves splicing a gene from fireflies into the TB bacteria as they grow. Resistant bacteria will actually glow in the dark; sensitive ones won't. Scientists are confident that the combination of breakthroughs such as these will eventually lead to the development of new and effective drugs to circumvent resistant tuberculosis bacteria and the knowledge to use them early enough in patient care to make a difference. But between now and that time the consequences of antibiotic-resistant bacteria could engulf the world with a plague unlike anything we've ever seen.

CHAPTER 4

The Possible Link Between Antibiotics and AIDS

Jim wasn't a patient of mine, but a friend of a friend, someone I met in 1984 at a social gathering. He asked if he could talk to me, and realizing that he was troubled, I said of course. We sat for over an hour in a quiet corner where Jim confessed to me that he was gay and had just left his wife to openly pursue a new life-style. Since 1984 was still relatively early in the AIDS epidemic, there was a great deal of superstition and conflicting information being disseminated by the media; even some of the most basic scientific facts were not yet clear. Jim was confused, frightened and eager for specific medical advice. I told him what I knew about the various risk factors, about safe sex and about other means of protecting himself.

A few weeks later, I heard from Jim again when he telephoned me at my office. He told me his internist was out of town for a week and wondered if I would mind terribly doing him a small favor. He described to me symptoms of a strep throat and asked if I could give him a prescription for an antibiotic. When I told him I would prefer to see him first in my office and take a specimen for throat culture, he told me he felt too ill to get out of bed. Besides, he said, he had had this before and knew what worked. There was no need to take up any more of my time. Somewhat reluctantly, I agreed to call in a prescription. Jim sounded relieved but wasn't yet finished giving me instructions. Expecting penicillin, the universal treatment for strep throat, he quickly volunteered that he was allergic to it and that erythromycin, the logical second choice, was no good either since it upset his stomach terribly. Tetracycline, he said, was what had worked for him in the past.

As impressed as I was with Jim's knowledge of the pharmacopeia, I was feeling increasingly uncomfortable with this conversation. But he was quite convincing and I gave in. After all, I rationalized, he wasn't asking for a controlled substance, just a simple antibiotic. I called his pharmacist and ordered forty tetracycline capsules. I was careful about specifying that no refills were to be given. I later found out that Jim had somehow persuaded the pharmacist to refill that tetracycline prescription four times in twelve months.

Over the next few years, I ran into Jim on several occasions, usually at recitals given by our mutual friend, a classical pianist. A recurrent pattern developed. Within a month or so after we saw each other, and did little more than exchange greetings, Jim would call me and ask for another antibiotic prescription, either tetracycline or one of the newer cephalosporins. The story changed a bit each time, but there was invariably a set of symptoms that seemed to require antibiotic therapy and Jim's internist was invariably out of town or otherwise unreachable. I finally resolved not to give in to him anymore. Apparently, he sensed I had been pushed to the limit, because he didn't call again.

In the spring of 1992, I was having lunch with our pianist friend and Jim's name came up. I hadn't seen or heard from him in over three years. When I asked about him, tears welled up in my friend's eyes as she told me that Jim had AIDS and was near death. He did, in fact, die within the month.

I agreed to accompany my friend to Jim's funeral. I now had some nagging questions, about Jim and about AIDS in general. The person I was hoping to see, Jim's internist, attended the funeral as well. I introduced myself and later we went to a nearby diner for coffee. I told him about the several telephone calls from Jim, and that I had allowed myself to be convinced by his stories. My colleague smiled sardonically and let me off the hook. He said that Jim was among the best manipulators he had seen, but the pattern of bargaining with physicians for antibiotics was extremely common among his gay patients. And this wasn't just his experience; it had happened to many other physicians.

I understood enough about the gay life-style to realize that antibiotic use was a natural consequence. The rate of treatable bacterial infections in this population, sexually transmitted and otherwise, was extremely high. Rather than be subjected to what they considered intense scrutiny and moralizing lectures, many gay men preferred to obfuscate the real reason for wanting the antibiotics.

It would have been easy just to let the matter rest there but I didn't. Operating partly on a hunch and partly on my background in immunology and pathology, I felt there was, just possibly, some link between the indiscriminate use of antibiotics and the mystery of AIDS. But I truly had no idea what it might be. The circuitous path I took from Jim's funeral to places as diverse as Berkeley, California; East Lansing, Michigan; Washington, D.C.; and Paris would lead me to a staggering hypothesis: the prolonged overuse of antibiotics to fight minor infections and to act as a general prophylaxis in the prevention of disease could, in fact, be contributing to the development of AIDS. Was this really possible? Could antibiotics be implicated as a contributing cause of AIDS? Was this crazy? As a matter of fact, it wasn't crazy at all. Some of the most highly regarded scientists in the world have come to that very conclusion.

The mobilization of the scientific community to fight AIDS was unprecedented. As a matter of fact, so great was our zeal to meet the challenge head-on that we may have been guilty of some sloppy science.

Just as law-enforcement agencies feel public pressure to apprehend the perpetrator when a series of vicious crimes is committed, so did the scientific community feel the necessity to identify the cause of acquired immune deficiency syndrome, or AIDS. Before a cure could be sought, a culprit had to be identified. And so, in the same way the police under these circumstances might collar an innocent bystander who looks suspicious, the medical community allowed itself to be swayed by circumstantial evidence.

Tissues of patients with this new disease were gone over with high-tech fine-tooth combs. Electron microscopes scanned for infectious particles or parts of infectious particles. Molecular amplification techniques and sophisticated immunochemistry screened for telltale new antibodies, signs that an infectious agent had been on the premises. And after having discarded several common viruses and bacteria as microbial red herrings, a group of scientists at the Institut Pasteur in Paris in 1983, led by Dr. Luc Montagnier, identified a novel viral particle that eventually came to be called the human immunodeficiency virus, or HIV. HIV belongs to a group of viruses known as retroviruses. These diabolical agents have a special ability to incorporate their own genes into those of cells they infect, thus commandeering the host genetic apparatus for their own purposes. In the case of HIV, the cells they primarily infect are in the immune system, specifically the T-cells. Specialized enzymes then direct the host cell to churn out new viral particles, which are assembled and leave the cell looking for new prey, and the cycle begins again.

The world was clamoring for the cause of AIDS, and HIV seemed to fill the bill. Medical judges and juries around the globe declared HIV guilty. The U.S. Secretary of Health and Human Services called a press conference and announced that the cause of AIDS had been identified. A cure would be just around the corner. Case closed.

Or was it? Once it became accepted that HIV was the cause of AIDS, most scientists were naturally swayed to make any subsequent data fit the HIV theory. But over the years, there have appeared too many cases that didn't fit the theory that HIV acted alone. Little by little there began to appear some cracks in the monolithic HIV-AIDS hypothesis.

Whether or not these chinks were intentionally kept from the public, most of us had no reason to question the apparently immutable HIV-AIDS connection until July 1992. Then, at the International AIDS Conference in Amsterdam, a small group of physicians abruptly turned the medical world on its ear by reporting thirty unusual cases of severe immunosuppression, or breakdown of the immune system. What was unusual was that each case appeared to be AIDS but all were HIV-negative. When this information was filtered and amplified by the media, it began to seem that a new mystery virus was on the loose. (One clever *Wall Street Journal* reporter, in a sarcastic derision of the alacrity with which some of his colleagues had jumped on this story, dubbed the as-yet-to-be-discovered new infectious agent MTV—"Media Transforming Virus.")

The fears of most of us were quieted, except for the one hundred or so patients identified within the next couple of months as having the same illness. After subsequent conferences at the World Health Organization in Geneva and the Centers for Disease Control and Prevention in Atlanta, experts confidently stated that there were no signs of a new epidemic and no signs of a new microbe.

This brought up a much larger and far more important question, one that was not answered by the experts. If it was indeed possible for a patient to develop a syndrome that so closely resembled and presented the same risks as AIDS without being infected with the HIV virus, just what was causing the immunosuppression? I was soon to meet scientists who had an intriguing answer. And I remembered an event five years earlier that now seemed particularly relevant.

In August 1987, my wife and I were spending the weekend with our close friends Dr. Charles Thomas and his wife at their summer home in Westport, Massachusetts, a place they had bought while Charlie was a professor of biochemistry at Harvard Medical School. Charlie showed me a paper that had been recently published in the journal *Cancer Research*. The paper had an innocent, even somewhat arcane-sounding, title, "Retroviruses as Carcinogens and Pathogens: Expectations and Reality." I knew, however, that this wasn't a modest paper. Charlie's gleaming eyes and his reputation for being a science contrarian contradicted that possibility.

The paper had been written by Peter H. Duesberg, a professor of molecular biology and virology at the University of California, Berkeley, and a recipient of an Outstanding Investigator Grant from the National Institutes of Health. Dr. Duesberg was and remains one of the world's most eminent authorities on retroviruses.

When I finished reading this dense twenty-page report, I was for the first time filled with doubts about whether HIV really was the cause of AIDS. In meticulous fashion, Dr. Duesberg had presented arguments and data refuting the conventional wisdom about HIV and AIDS. If one subscribed to the tenets of good science, he claimed, there was no other conclusion that could be drawn other than that HIV was most definitely *not* the cause of AIDS.

For one thing, he wrote, the long latent period of AIDS following HIV infection was inconsistent with the known behavior of the virus. In the test tube, HIV multiplies within several days, much like any other retrovirus. And even in humans, infection is followed by an antibody response within four to seven weeks. By contrast, the lag between infection and the appearance of AIDS is estimated to take years. In his 1987 paper, Duesberg said there was no logical explanation that incorporated HIV as the cause. In addition, he said, if HIV were killing susceptible T-cells, one would expect both to find high levels of virus in the T-cells of AIDS patients and to be able to demonstrate in the laboratory that HIV was capable of such a killing effect once it entered the cells. According to Duesberg, neither is this the case. In only 15 percent of AIDS patients was virus identified at all, and even in those cases, HIV is found in only one cell in ten thousand, not consistent with the devastation seen in AIDS. For these reasons (and some others more esoteric), Dr. Duesberg believed HIV was merely another red herring. Although in this paper he didn't address what he thought was the cause, he pointed out that by putting all our eggs in the HIV basket, we were wasting precious time and resources.

Duesberg's arguments were a stunning antithesis to what virtually all the world had accepted as an ironclad truth for more than four years. Could it be that the emperor really had no clothes? Most scientists in the AIDS field I asked dismissed Duesberg's theories and him with a wave and a grimace. I never did know whether I received these responses because the disease had become so politicized that by even questioning the HIV-AIDS hypothesis one risked being ostracized from the research community, or because Dr. Duesberg had a grating, polemical manner that tended to turn people off, or because the weight of evidence truly wasn't convincing. In any case, the whole issue lay dormant—punctured only by occasional jabs from Dr. Duesberg, mostly in the popular press—until 1992 and the Amsterdam conference.

It was then I decided I had to do my own journalistic research and discuss this with Dr. Duesberg. During our several conversations on the telephone and in his office on the magnificent Berkeley campus, although Duesberg was gracious and helpful, it was obvious he had not shed the ready-for-battle posture that had clearly muddied his message. He was as resolute as ever in his opinion that HIV was not the cause of AIDS. His position was now so extreme that he no longer believed that AIDS was the result of an infection at all. Furthermore, he now believed he "knew" the cause. It was drugs, he said. Intravenous drugs, psychoactive drugs (especially cocaine) and amazingly even AZT, the first drug approved for the *treatment* of the disease. All these compounds, according to Duesberg, are powerful immunosuppressants, much more powerful than the HIV virus itself, which he called a puny pathogen.

This was all tantalizing, but he hadn't mentioned antibiotics, the subject in which I was mainly interested, in his list of drugs. Did they belong somewhere on the spectrum? Definitely, answered Dr. Duesberg, but he admitted to not being expert in their effects on the immune system. For that, he referred me to another scientist, Dr. Robert Root-Bernstein. Although I had found Duesberg intriguing, I was happy to be directed elsewhere. It seemed to me that, in completely dismissing HIV as having a role in AIDS, he was guilty of being as intransigent as those he criticized.

Dr. Robert Root-Bernstein is a physiologist and immunologist at Michigan State University and has a much cooler head than Peter Duesberg. He clearly agreed with many points Duesberg made, but took a position far less extreme. In the first of several conversations I had with him, we talked about the HIV-free cases of AIDS, and he told me those that had been reported in Amsterdam were not new. They had been reported in the medical literature since 1986. The number of these cases, Dr. Root-Bernstein said, was highly significant, and there were many more than the hundred or so we had come to know about by the end of 1992. He also told me that, as early as 1989, the Centers for Disease Control reported that 5 percent of all AIDS patients in the United States who had been tested for HIV to that time were HIV-negative. That would be well over one thousand people. As of late 1992, when he told me this, the statistics had not yet been updated. Had they been, the number would have undoubtedly swelled even more.

This, Root-Bernstein pointed out, was central to what I was looking for. "The existence of HIV-free AIDS proves that HIV is not a necessary cause of acquired immunodeficiency," he said. He also said, however, that "this does not preclude HIV from playing some role in most AIDS cases, but it may also mean that HIV is not the primary immunosuppressive agent in AIDS. The public acknowledgement of HIV-free AIDS makes it untenable not to reconsider the idea that these agents are themselves sufficient to cause AIDS." So, by itself, HIV in his opinion did not create the disease.

When I asked him about the possibility of another causative virus and the failure of scientists around the world to find it, he said he was not the least bit surprised. Given the amount of work done on HIV over the past decade, he said, the possibility that a new lymphotropic virus (a virus with an affinity for the immune cells) had been overlooked by almost every laboratory in the world was remote. Root-Bernstein told me it was "much more likely that HIV-free AIDS cases are due to known causes of immunosuppression that have not previously been considered significant by mainstream researchers."

The known causes of immunosuppression he was referring to came under the general category of cofactors, or helpers. Under this theory, if HIV infection is in fact involved in AIDS, the virus may not be able to cause AIDS itself. It needs serious help to take the condition from infection to life-threatening disease. And, in some cases, the cofactors may become the primary factors, able to cause AIDS without the need for HIV infection at all. The cofactors, Root-Bernstein said, definitely included antibiotics. He had a great interest in that topic, as well as a large file of literature. He promised to send it off to me right away. After I read it, we would get together again and discuss his information in detail.

In the meantime, with the notion of cofactors in general and antibiotics in particular now firmly fixed in my mind, I sought an interview with the discoverer of the HIV virus, Dr. Luc Montagnier of the Pasteur Institute in Paris, thinking he would be the most avid proponent of the HIV-acting-alone theory. But like all great scientists, Dr. Montagnier was open-minded. In a 1992 issue of the British scientific journal *Nature,* the editor, John Maddux, wrote the following: "Montagnier said clearly what he meant. HIV is a necessary but not, without the cofactor, a sufficient cause of AIDS." Montagnier had made that statement in May 1992, at the alternative AIDS conference, also held in Amsterdam. He repeated it two months later at the International AIDS Conference.

After reading that comment in *Nature,* I wanted to find out more about Dr. Montagnier's concept of cofactors. With a dear friend from Lausanne, Switzerland, acting as a French-speaking intermediary (although Professor Montagnier speaks English fluently, his staff does not and I speak no French), we set up an appointment in September 1992. My friend told me she had been warned in advance by his assistants that this was an even busier time than usual for Dr. Montagnier. What with the HIV-without-AIDS story breaking in July and Dr. Montagnier's claim that HIV may need cofactors in order to cause AIDS, the disease and its most famous researcher were more in the news than ever. He was in constant demand and would be able to spare only a few moments.

How wrong his assistants were. In a manner as relaxed as Dr. Duesberg's was frenetic, Luc Montagnier spent more than one hour on the telephone with me, describing in great detail how he came upon the idea that cofactors were necessary and how he viewed them as involved with AIDS. This was clearly a concept for which Dr. Montagnier had great passion.

But Dr. Montagnier is a careful scientist and did not want to be in any way misinterpreted. He began by making certain I understood that HIV cofactor theories in general were still very much in the minority. "The vast majority of scientists still believe that HIV acting alone is both necessary and sufficient to cause AIDS," he said. But he and a growing segment of other researchers in the field believe that while HIV is necessary, it is not by itself capable of causing AIDS. In addition, his specific notion of the predominant cofactor was still very much a hypothesis. Although he had both laboratory and epidemiological data to back up his theory, he was not yet ready to state unequivocally that this is what happens.

Once he laid the ground rules, however, he led me on a remarkable journey that clearly linked antibiotic use with AIDS, and in a way I hadn't expected at all. As with so many extraordinary scientific discoveries, Dr. Montagnier's was serendipitous.

In 1990, he and his colleagues were testing potential alternatives to the drug AZT, not because they agreed with Dr. Duesberg that it could actually cause AIDS (there are few things about Duesberg's theories that struck a responsive chord in Luc Montagnier), but because it was far from a perfect treatment. Although several studies had reported that AZT had improved the clinical and immunological status of patients with AIDS and AIDS-related complex, administration of the drug was often associated with severe toxicity, particularly bone marrow suppression.

In the course of his search for anti-HIV compounds, Dr. Montagnier observed something startling: that the common antibiotic tetracycline was able to inhibit the cell-killing effect of HIV in a laboratory test tube. He then found the same result with HIV-2, the other recognized viral cause of AIDS. This was clearly an unforeseen phenomenon that needed further study, since antibiotics have no impact on viruses at all. It was the next set of experiments that led to the breakthrough.

Montagnier and his colleagues tested again and, of course, found that protection against the killing effect of HIV was not at all accompanied by inhibition of virus production. There was no way it could be. The antibiotic wasn't inhibiting growth of the HIV virus, but it *was* inhibiting cell damage. This had to mean that the antibiotic was successfully working on something else. And whatever that was, was the culprit. The very same group of French scientists that only seven years earlier had discovered HIV were now faced with the fascinating and perplexing question: What was that something else? The cofactor had to be bacterial.

The most likely possibility, they decided, was that a tetracycline-sensitive organism was playing a role as a cofactor in HIV-induced cell death. After ruling out a wide array of bacteria, they came upon a type of organism called *Mycoplasma* as the most likely candidate. Mycoplasmas are the smallest microorganisms capable of independent replication and growth, in many ways a cross between bacteria and viruses. When Montagnier was then able to actually isolate *Mycoplasma* from HIV cells growing in the laboratory, his suspicions became much stronger that he was onto something big.

But he immediately met with criticism. This had all taken place in vitro, in the laboratory, not in the real world of AIDS patients. "In vitro, many infectious agents interact with HIV," said Dr. Jerome Groopman of the New England Deaconess Hospital, a recognized authority on AIDS and a leading proponent of the HIV-acting-alone theory. According to him it was an interesting observation but without clinical relevance. Other scientists pointed out that *Mycoplasma* was a ubiquitous organism and a frequent contaminant of cell cultures. It might very well be just another red herring.

But Montagnier was undaunted in his belief that the *Mycoplasma* phenomenon was real. AIDS is characterized primarily by a profound alteration in the function and number of T-lymphocytes, specifically those T-cells known as CD4. The belief, originally advanced by Montagnier along with others, is that this is the result of infection with HIV. But, as Dr. Montagnier explained to me, although several hypotheses have been proposed over the past decade to explain the specific cell killing associated with HIV infection, none of them— including some of his own, he admitted—is sufficient to explain completely the extensive cell destruction that occurs in AIDS patients. The theories have also not been able to account adequately for the wide variation in the length of time of disease incubation following HIV infection and the rapidity of disease progression. Therefore, he and his colleagues were convinced something else must be involved, namely *Mycoplasma*. (Here is where Montagnier and Duesberg do have some accord in their thinking. Although the two came to different conclusions about AIDS, it was their recognition of similar inconsistencies in the HIV theory that led them to question the conventional wisdom.)

Confidence in Montagnier's theory was buoyed shortly thereafter, and some of his loudest critics were muted, when his group announced they had detected *Mycoplasma* in live patients with AIDS—in homosexuals, intravenous drug users and transfusion recipients—for the first time. They found evidence of *Mycoplasma* infection in 37 of 97 patients with AIDS, and were actually able to isolate the organisms in 16 of the 37. Contrasted with finding *Mycoplasma* in only 1 of 20 healthy controls, they knew this was no artifact.

If *Mycoplasma* was, indeed, a necessary cofactor in AIDS and it continued to live in the body in the same way in which it was observed in the test tube, it could be killed by tetracycline and we would have a cure for AIDS. But the grim paradox was that continued use of the antibiotic transformed the *Mycoplasma* in the body into a related but sufficiently different organism—a microsphere—which could not be killed by tetracycline.

The story of this drug-resistant organism began with the sexual revolution of the 1960s and 1970s. It is well documented that during that time there was a dramatic increase in the incidence of sexually transmitted disease, and hence a concomitant increase in the use of antibiotics to treat these conditions. The drug that was perhaps used most commonly was tetracycline, a broad-spectrum antibiotic. It was effective against a variety of conditions, such as gonorrhea and chlamydial infection. But when antibiotics are taken, they affect not only the organisms they are intended to kill but innocent bystanders as well. Mycoplasmas, Dr. Montagnier believes, were such innocent bystanders. Although they were known to occasionally cause a pneumonia, for the most part mycoplasmas were relatively harmless microorganisms that populated our bodies. And with the excessive use of antibiotics, although still harmless, many strains of *Mycoplasma* became tetracycline-resistant.

As this practice of excessive antibiotic use continued in the 1980s, the already drug-resistant mycoplasmas continued to change. One thing that happened is that previously rare species of *Mycoplasma*, especially those known as *Mycoplasma pirium* and *Mycoplasma fermentans*, began to grow in the bodies of gay males who took large amounts of antibiotics. They were especially prone to populate the urinary tracts of these people.

Another change, one very important in the theory of how antibiotics and *Mycoplasma* came to be cofactors in AIDS, is that these new strains underwent a structural metamorphosis. Only a few weeks before I spoke with Dr. Montagnier he had discovered something that had never before been seen in these bacteria. He found that *Mycoplasma fermentans* can exist in two different forms in its life cycle. One is the normal or filamentous form, but the other, the new form, was called microspheres by Dr. Montagnier. As their name implies, they are tiny, round submicroscopic particles, which contain all the genetic material of the larger filamentous form but which are so small and compact that they can get inside the T-cells, the same cells infected by HIV. This was unheard of for bacteria, even primitive bacteria such as *Mycoplasma,* which are generally thousands of times larger than viruses. Living inside the cell was until then the private domain of viruses.

Once the microspheres are inside the T-lymphocytes, there is a variety of scenarios that can take place. And one of these is an interaction with HIV to trigger the progression from infection to full-blown AIDS. How does this happen? One way could be through acting as intracellular nurses, providing more "food" for the HIV, something the HIV is unable to do for itself. By merely infecting the T-cells, the *Mycoplasma* would stimulate them to release growth-promoting substances called cytokines. These cytokines, in turn, stimulate the maturation of more of the type of T-cells that HIV needs to attack, thereby allowing it to multiply and cause destruction.

This scenario wasn't depicted to me by Dr. Montagnier but instead by Dr. Joseph Tully of the National Institutes of Allergy and Infectious Disease. Although not an expert on AIDS, Dr. Tully is considered by many the leading scholar on *Mycoplasma* in the United States. Dr. Montagnier believes this may in fact happen to some extent. But he doesn't think this is the main way *Mycoplasma* and HIV interact. The growth-factor stimulation, he said, occurs with virtually all infections, and if it played a prominent role in the triggering of HIV-infected cells to progress to AIDS, other infections would do it regularly as well. This has not been demonstrated.

What happens specifically between *Mycoplasma* and HIV, Montagnier believes, is the following. He has recently developed evidence that many HIV particles are structurally defective. Rather than acting as nurses and providing food for the HIV, the mycoplasmas instead act as microbial repairmen by producing a series of essential proteins that the HIV is missing, proteins it needs to grow. The specific proteins had just been identified by Dr. Montagnier when I spoke to him. In fact, he said, this work was so new in September 1992 that he and his colleagues hadn't yet even submitted it for publication to a scientific journal. By providing these proteins, the drug-resistant mycoplasmas give a remarkable boost to HIV replication, leading to the extensive cell destruction and death characteristic of AIDS. Since those who are already infected with HIV are quite prone to becoming infected with antibiotic-resistant *Myco-plasma fermentans,* Montagnier believes this is the main cofactor role these bacteria play.

Then he told me there are other ways in which the antibiotic-resistant *Mycoplasma* can accomplish a progression to AIDS as well. He had discovered that the microspheres of *Mycoplasma fermen-tans* are themselves immunosuppressive agents, even in the absence of HIV. There are many instances, Dr. Montagnier feels, in which the mycoplasmas are the first invader. Once having done this, in most instances the microspheres cause a mild level of immunosup-pression and then sit dormant inside the T-cells, waiting for their coconspirator, HIV, to come along. And this often happens because the mild immunosuppression makes those infected with the *Myco-plasma* more vulnerable to subsequent infection with HIV. The havoc then begins.

In some cases, however, the mycoplasmas turn aggressive without waiting for HIV. Rather than just cause mild immunosuppression, they cause severe immunosuppression, an actual progression to AIDS. Just as the CDC and the WHO concluded, Dr. Montagnier doesn't believe there is another virus involved in the cases of AIDS without HIV. Unlike them, however, he believes he has the answer, and that answer is *Mycoplasma fermentans* acting alone. Why did no other scientists find these bacteria when they were looking? Dr. Montagnier's answer, given with the confidence of a scientist who has tasted major success before, is that mycoplasmas are very deli-cate organisms and difficult to detect. If they had looked more care-fully, he said, they would have found them.

Even while the work of the members of the Pasteur Institute team was in its early stages, they already had an ally in the United States, but it wasn't until Montagnier published his findings that the two scientists got together to compare notes. Several years earlier, in 1986, Shyh-Ching Lo, a young virologist and pathologist, claimed to have discovered a "novel virus" in tumor cells taken from AIDS pa-tients with Kaposi's sarcoma. Although he was excoriated in meet-ings by other virologists for reporting without sufficient data, Dr. Lo, who did his original work at the National Cancer Institute but, when I spoke with him, was chief of the division of molecular patho-biology at the Armed Forces Institute of Pathology in Washington,

D.C., pressed on. He later admitted he had made a mistake in dubbing what he had found a new viral particle, but it was no mistake that he had found something. That "something" turned out to be *Mycoplasma;* and after several exchanges of data, both Dr. Lo and Dr. Montagnier confirmed to me that it was highly likely they were working on the same phenomenon, the intracellular microspheres of *Mycoplasma* which resulted from antibiotic-induced transformation.

Not only did what was being found in the laboratory and in patients provide a solid foundation for Dr. Montagnier's hypothesis, but he then also painted a vivid picture for me which would explain many of the epidemiological inconsistencies regarding AIDS. Although he again stressed to me that this is still a theory, it fits very well with what has happened. The same cannot be said for the prevailing wisdom.

With what is accepted at present, we cannot explain the development of AIDS solely on the basis of HIV. Although AIDS is a relatively new disease, it is well accepted now that HIV has existed for many decades in Africa without causing any problems. Somehow, it eventually was transformed into a virus with a higher infectivity, enough to cause AIDS.

When this happened, the conventional wisdom goes, the virus came from Africa to the United States, and the AIDS epidemic began. But this is as far as these theories go, and they are full of holes. One of the main inconsistencies, Montagnier said, is that the AIDS epidemic didn't begin solely in the United States, but also in Africa, at approximately the same time as in the United States. And, contrary to popular belief, the early AIDS cases in Africa were not in rural areas but in the big cities in Zaire and Zimbabwe.

What Dr. Montagnier believes happened instead, which fits with these data, is that antibiotic-resistant *Mycoplasma* developed in American homosexuals overdosing on antibiotics in the late 1970s. These mycoplasmas were then carried to Africa, where they mixed with HIV, and that is how the AIDS epidemic began. This alone explains the transformation of the HIV virus into a destructive form. As more HIV was brought back to New York, San Francisco and other large American cities, there was further interaction with the antibiotic-resistant *Mycoplasma* that was waiting there. Haiti, where many of the early AIDS cases were seen, was a country caught in the middle. It is well documented, Montagnier told me, that many Haitians traveled to Africa during the 1960s and 1970s. They could easily have brought back HIV with them, which remained dormant until they were infected with the antibiotic-resistant *Mycoplasma* by American tourists.

CHAPTER 5

Completing the AIDS Hypothesis

When I spoke again with Dr. Root-Bernstein, I was to discover that there was another path between antibiotics and AIDS, one just as interesting and even more direct. It didn't in any way conflict with what I had learned from Montagnier but rather embellished it.

Whereas Luc Montagnier's research implicates antibiotic use as a catalytic agent in the development of AIDS, Robert Root-Bernstein maintains that antibiotic use can contribute directly to the development of the disease. The difference between these points of view is essentially a matter of emphasis. The ways in which their concepts overlap only strengthen the argument that links antibiotics with AIDS.

Dr. Montagnier, the discoverer of HIV, has not changed his mind about the presence of HIV being essential to AIDS. When, at the Eighth International AIDS Conference in Amsterdam in July 1992, he said, "I think we should put the same weight on the cofactors as we have on HIV," he stated his position clearly. He no longer believed HIV was sufficient to cause AIDS but still felt it was necessary, although he does grant that there can be exceptions to the involvement of HIV.

Dr. Root-Bernstein, on the other hand, has deliberately chosen to stay outside the established thinking about HIV and AIDS. He is on the editorial board of a newly formed group in San Francisco, "Re-thinking AIDS." Organized by Dr. Charles Thomas, it is composed of several respected scientists who are calling for a reappraisal of the existing hypothesis that HIV is the cause of AIDS. They are developing a hypothesis that may not include HIV at all.

Root-Bernstein believes that HIV is just another immune-suppressing cofactor. He began his second meeting with me by explaining why he felt that cofactors played a significant role in AIDS. He was originally drawn to this concept in much the same way Dr. Montagnier and Dr. Duesberg were, by observing that it is virtually impossible for an infection caused by a single virus with affinity for T-lymphocytes to simultaneously suppress all the different components of the immune system, as is characteristic of AIDS patients: T-cells, natural killer cells, B-cells and macrophages. This, along with the increasing rate of AIDS cases without HIV, made Root-Bernstein highly suspicious that there must be something other than HIV involved.

And recent epidemiological data clinched it for him. Studies of gay men and intravenous drug abusers show that the average time from infection to overt AIDS is ten years. If HIV alone controlled AIDS, he said, then about half of the people infected with HIV in 1983 should have developed AIDS by 1993. Yet this is not true of hemophiliacs, a well-defined group that is easy to study. Of the 15,000 hemophiliacs in the United States who were infected with HIV between 1981 and 1984, one would expect at least half of them to have developed AIDS by now. Yet only 1,500 cases of AIDS among hemophiliacs—10 percent of those infected—have been recorded during the entire epidemic. "If anything proves that HIV alone does not control the development of AIDS, this is it," Root-Bernstein said.

So what else is involved? "Before we can accept HIV as the sole cause of immunosuppression, he said, "it is necessary to assure ourselves that alternative explanations of the data do not exist." In other words, we must determine that the HIV theory is necessary and sufficient to explain AIDS and that no other theory is necessary or sufficient. In this regard, a crucial question is: Do AIDS patients have any identified immunosuppressive risks other than HIV?

The answer, he said, is a definite yes. "All AIDS patients do have multiple causes of immunosuppression prior to, concomitant with, subsequent to and sometimes even in the absence of HIV infection." These immunosuppressive agents are of seven basic types: chronic or repeated infectious diseases caused by immunosuppressive organisms (*Mycoplasma* falls into this category); recreational and addictive drugs; anesthetics; semen components; blood (from intravenous drug use and transfusions); malnutrition; and antibiotics. While few AIDS patients are likely to encounter all of these agents, Root-Bernstein's research has demonstrated that all encounter at least one of them and very likely several.

Antibiotic abuse, he said, is an immunosuppressive factor that has been particularly overlooked as a risk factor for developing AIDS. There is a sad irony here. In contrast to every other item on the cofactor list, antibiotics are viewed as a disease preventive. The evidence is strong that they may be doing just the opposite.

Antibiotic abuse is especially common in the two largest population groups at risk for AIDS: gay men and intravenous drug users. Gay men were aware of their disease vulnerability long before AIDS emerged as a problem. Many of them readily volunteered for tests of experimental hepatitis vaccines in the 1970s. Many became chronic users of antibiotics, either prophylactically or to treat recurrent venereal infections and other problems. Antibiotics are almost always self-administered and frequently obtained by manipulating unsuspecting physicians and even pharmacists.

A formal survey of antibiotic use among gay men was published in 1987 in the *Southern Medical Journal*. Dr. Linda Pifer and her associates at the University of Tennessee School of Medicine conducted an extensive study of regular male homosexual patrons of gay bars in Memphis. Along with other overlapping practices, such as the abuse of recreational drugs and the routine use of inhalant nitrites, more than 40 percent of the men were found to be regularly treating themselves with prescription antibiotics.

Many intravenous drug users are also aware of their unusual risk of infection and therefore also take prophylactic measures that they believe protect them. In a letter to the editor in the *Journal of the American Medical Association*, Drs. Scott R. and Sydria K. Schaffer, who practice internal medicine in Philadelphia, reported that approximately 60 percent of the intravenous drug abusers they saw during a three-month period at the emergency rooms of Temple University and Hahnemann University hospitals were using antibiotics in the hope of preventing cellulitis, phlebitis and abscess formation, all common infections in intravenous drug abusers.

The feeling of these physicians was that considerably more than 60 percent were using antibiotics. A good reason for withholding this information from the interviewers was to conceal the way in which the antibiotics were frequently obtained. Virtually every one of the IV drug abusers seen by these doctors admitted that they received antibiotics on the street from their drug dealer.

Antibiotic abuse and illicit drug abuse have become synonymous, a practice repeated daily for months or even years on end. "The irony of the situation," Dr. Root-Bernstein said, "is that in protecting themselves against everyday infections, they open themselves up to more exotic and more deadly infections." Many of these infections, such as *Pneumocystis* pneumonia, fall under the umbrella of the almost thirty conditions currently defined as AIDS.

The most common antibiotic supplied, reported by every patient the Philadelphia doctors saw who admitted to antibiotic abuse, was the cephalosporin Keflex, a broad-spectrum antibiotic. Besides fostering the development of bacterial resistance, Keflex also has strong immunosuppressive properties. This is not merely a theoretical risk; the connection has been demonstrated clinically. Dr. P. H. Chandrasekar and his colleagues at Wayne State University School of Medicine in Detroit reported in 1990 that illicit antibiotic use was one of the main factors (along with the duration of intravenous drug use, sexual promiscuity, and malnutrition) closely associated with the subsequent development of AIDS. In many cases, the association was completely independent of infection with HIV.

Antibiotics have been recognized as immune-suppressing substances for some time. As far back as the 1950s, in the still early days of antibiotic use, there were many reports published that high doses of penicillin compounds often resulted in opportunistic infections with various fungi and yeasts, such as *Candida albicans*. Although elimination of the yeast's enemies—the so-called good bacteria—by the antibiotic plays a role in these infections, so does an impairment in our body's immune system, whose function is to stop these ubiquitous organisms from overgrowing. Yeast infections have ranged from the annoying but nonthreatening vaginal variety to the deadly *Candida* septicemias increasingly common in cancer and AIDS patients.

This immune impairment occurs through a variety of biochemical mechanisms, depending on the drug involved. The antibiotic chloramphenicol is described as "immunotoxic" because it has been established that it can inhibit several types of immune responses, sometimes quite severely. When men previously immunized for tetanus were given chloramphenicol for ten to fourteen days and then given a booster injection, their antibody response—which should have been vigorous—was actually significantly suppressed. It has even been possible for researchers to prolong the survival of skin grafts between completely unrelated donor and recipient animals by giving the recipient chloramphenicol in advance to prevent the immune system's rejection. This was not a welcome discovery with potential therapeutic implications for human transplantation, but rather an indication of how broad the repressive reach of this antibiotic is across the entire immune spectrum. The most widely accepted account of how chloramphenicol is able to so effectively suppress immune function is that it is very efficient at inhibiting all protein synthesis, including the proteins the immune system needs to perform its various tasks.

If this effect were limited to chloramphenicol, there would be little danger for gays, IV drug users and others at risk for contracting AIDS. Chloramphenicol, however, is only the prototype for a wide range of antibiotics that have a suppressive effect on protein synthesis and therefore on several aspects of immunity. The mechanisms differ slightly from drug to drug but they all work in much the same way. Most notable among this group is tetracycline, the antibiotic Luc Montagnier correlated with the resistant *Mycoplasma* when he proposed a different way its use can lead to AIDS. Tetracycline is a favorite of gay men as a prophylactic drug.

Other antibiotics, those that interfere with the metabolism of folic acid, are potentially dangerous to immunity as well. Included in this group are the sulfa drugs, as well as trimethoprim and pyrimethamine. Inhibition of folic acid synthesis is beneficial to a point, since bacteria need to make this vitamin in order to reproduce. But if the antibiotic is taken for long periods of time, or in high doses, its effects go beyond inhibition of microbes and interfere with immunology.

Many of the newer antibiotics, including the latest cephalosporins (which the Philadelphia survey found were abused by every one of the intravenous drug users interviewed), amikacin and piperacillin, have been described as "immunomodulatory," meaning that they affect only specific parts of the immune system, implying that they are less devastating. In terms of progression toward AIDS, however, that is not the case. A part of the immune system these antibiotics do modify is the T-cells, the area that most goes awry in AIDS.

How do they do this? It has been demonstrated that the antibiotics in this group deplete or bind and otherwise make unavailable crucial minerals, especially zinc but also calcium and selenium. T-cells are known to require one or more of these elements for division and cloning, necessary components of an immune response to a foreign invader. Lacking this ability, one would quickly become vulnerable to the type of opportunistic infections characteristic of AIDS. In 1992 scientists at Vanderbilt University School of Medicine discovered that the subset of T-cells that require zinc for growth the most are those known as CD4, a term which by now has become familiar in the AIDS vocabulary. By definition, AIDS cannot exist without a depletion of CD4 T-cells below a level of 300.

Even without using antibiotics, gay men and IV drug users typically have unusually low serum levels of zinc and selenium compared with heterosexual men and women and lesbians. Although the reason for this hasn't been determined conclusively, some scientists believe it secondary to poor nutrition, increased numbers of infections, or a combination of the two. This has been found in completely asymptomatic individuals, not just those already diagnosed with AIDS. So, when you add antibiotic use, you are adding something that severely exacerbates any already existing nutritional deficiencies, further compromises the immune system and pushes it over the brink.

Antibiotics specifically used to treat parasitic infections also have a variety of immunosuppressive effects. Africans could be especially affected by these drugs. Prone to both malaria and a parasitic worm infestation called schistosomiasis, Africans also show a proneness to develop AIDS. Chloroquine, the antibiotic most commonly used to treat or prevent malaria, has been extensively studied for its immunosuppressive effects. In laboratory studies, the proliferation of T-cells, as well as their ability to kill foreign invaders, was decreased from 25 to 100 percent after treatment with chloroquine. So potent an immunosuppressive agent is chloroquine that it is even occasionally used in the treatment of severe rheumatoid arthritis, a disease manifested by excessive activity of the immune system, in many ways on the opposite end of the spectrum from AIDS. According to Dr. Root-Bernstein, there have not been any adequate studies under clinical conditions of the immunological toxicity of antiparasitic drugs, but it is his feeling that they are involved in the high incidence of AIDS in Africa.

Gay men use antiparasitic antibiotics extensively. From 20 to 50 percent of gay men in major American cities experience repeated bouts of the "gay bowel syndrome," a confluence of several parasitic infections (such as amebiasis and giardiasis) in their intestinal tract. Because of this, they are routinely treated (even prophylactically by themselves and by some physicians) with antiparasitic antibiotics.

There are still other ways in which antibiotics could conceivably increase the development of AIDS, some through the immune system and others via different mechanisms. The antifungal drug ketoconazole, often used to treat infections of gay men at risk for AIDS, inhibits the production of cortisol by the adrenal gland and subsequently causes loss of appetite, weight loss, potassium and sodium disturbances in the blood, as well as low blood pressure. Lack of adrenal cortisol reserve is extremely dangerous for anyone subjected to major stress, especially surgery.

The antibiotic rifampin accelerates the breakdown of adrenal cortisone. The antibiotic trimethoprim-sulfamethoxazole, commonly used by gays and IV drug users, has been associated with acute pancreatitis, a condition found in half of gay men on autopsy. This is the same antibiotic that has an adverse effect on folic acid.

Nitrite compounds are not antibiotics but can interact with them in an evil way. Inhalants such as amyl nitrite and butyl nitrite, more commonly known as "poppers" or "snappers," are mainstays of the gay life-style. The same study on gay men in Memphis which found that 40 percent regularly abused antibiotics also reported that 80 percent of the men used nitrite compounds at least occasionally and that 30 percent used them more than once a week. In major cities such as Washington, D.C., San Francisco, Los Angeles and New York, approximately 95 percent of gay men report using nitrites, often regularly. The reason for abusing these drugs relates to the dilatory effect they have on smooth muscles throughout the body. This facilitates anal intercourse and, because of the dilation of blood vessels in the brain, apparently enhances sexual pleasure.

Nitrite compounds themselves have an immunosuppressive effect, and early on in the AIDS epidemic the Centers for Disease Control seriously considered the possibility that nitrite abuse was the cause of AIDS. (This was before the discovery of HIV.) Especially frightening is the prospect of what can happen when nitrites and antibiotics are taken together, a highly likely occurrence since abuse of both drugs is extremely common. In the test tube and in animal studies, it has been shown that nitrites can convert most antibiotics into carcinogens; and although not yet proven, it has been suggested that this same chemical reaction may occur in many gay men. If that were true, it could account for the unusually high incidence of both Kaposi's sarcoma and lymphoma (cancer of the lymph nodes) that is found almost uniquely in this risk group.

Where, then, does all this information leave us? No matter what we have believed up until now, we have to be suspicious of the role of HIV in the development of AIDS. Since we have become so accustomed to calling it "the virus that causes AIDS" or even equating HIV infection with having AIDS, it will be difficult to revise our thinking. But it is clearly time for us to focus on the cofactors, especially antibiotics. The scientific literature on the immune-suppressing effects of antibiotics is too abundant to be ignored. This message must be disseminated to all those at risk.

CHAPTER 6

Dangerous Exports from the Third World

When Marshall McLuhan called the world a global village, he was describing the outcome of an electronic revolution. That phrase can now be applied to antibiotic resistance. The global village has, in fact, become a test tube for breeding a multitude of antibiotic-resistant strains of microorganisms. The United States and the rest of the industrialized world have done a poor job of dealing with this problem. But even with a well-conceived plan that was perfectly implemented, we would still be in trouble. The amount of antibiotic-resistant bacteria spewed into the environment in the developed world is a mere trickle compared with the torrent flooding the Third World.

The consequences we face as a result of this Third World dilemma are not hypothetical exercises for scientists to ponder in the medical literature. It is a grave problem that has the potential to affect us as directly as any foreign crisis we see on television or read about in the newspapers. It is a dilemma without national or political boundaries.

Just as these potentially lethal bacteria gain strength in our hospitals and are then disseminated into the community, so do the resistant bacteria selected for in Nigeria or Chile or Thailand add to an expanding global pool. The fallout created can eventually reverberate throughout the entire world. With nowhere to hide, none of us will be able to find protection from bacteria that have become as common and dangerous an export from developing countries as cocaine and heroin, which we have been just as unsuccessful in interdicting.

Global travel is what connects us to antibiotic resistance in the Third World. Bacteria that develop there easily attach themselves to visitors or to products and hitch a ride across oceans and continents. There are many reasons why the Third World provides such fertile soil for the production of resistant bacteria. Some are cultural, some economic. But it finally comes down to two basic factors: inappropriate antibiotics and inappropriate doses. These are at the heart of our problem in the industrialized world as well. But in the developing world they take on a truly bizarre aspect.

Sjaak van der Geest, a Dutch medical anthropologist, describes an experience he had at the Central Lorrystation of Kumasi in Ghana. Shortly after he arrived, his attention was caught by a young boy hawking capsules from a plastic bag. Dr. van der Geest asked what the capsules were for. "Piles," answered the boy with an air of authority.

Van der Geest followed the boy around the station, watching for some time as he plied his wares. Later, he saw the boy sell the pills as a cure for sexual impotence. His curiosity piqued, van der Geest finally bought this wonder drug himself, paying two and a half shillings for a single capsule. When he arrived back in Holland, he had the drug analyzed. It turned out to be Penbritin, 250 milligrams. Penbritin is an antibiotic, certainly useful in the treatment of susceptible bacterial infections, but hardly indicated for treating piles, sexual impotence, or whatever other ailments the entrepreneurial boy sold the antibiotic for that day.

In the open markets in Nairobi and most other African cities, an array of antibiotic capsules is displayed on huge trays alongside equally colorful sweets and candies. On any given day, one can see long lines of people waiting to buy a single capsule of chloramphenicol or tetracycline or penicillin to self-medicate a headache or a stomach pain or sometimes not to treat a disease at all, but merely as a blanket protection against venereal disease. Weaving throughout these same markets are vendors hustling antibiotics the same way New York City street vendors sell watches, T-shirts and incense.

Taking one capsule wouldn't do much, but hundreds of thousands of people in the Third World regularly buy antibiotics from street vendors as part of their daily routine.

These are perfect setups for danger. Every time an uncontrolled use of antibiotics like this occurs, there is a selection of resistant strains, either of pathogenic bacteria (if any happen to be present) or of friendly bacteria, which are always present. That's why there is a much greater prevalence of ampicillin resistance, for example, in Vellore, India, than in Edinburgh, Scotland, and why in Kenya, most strains of *E. coli* bacteria isolated from stools in a pediatric observation ward were resistant to streptomycin, tetracycline and ampicillin, and why in Bangladesh, more than 80 percent of *Shigella* bacteria are resistant to ampicillin and trimethoprim, the first agents recommended in the treatment of dysentery.

In another study on children, this time on perfectly healthy children, there was a comparison made among the intestinal bacteria of infants and small children from Boston, Caracas, Venezuela, and Qin Pu, China. The study specifically looked at how resistant were the intestinal bacteria in children who had never taken any antibiotic (That it was difficult to find children from any of the locations in this category, even though they were all under five years old, is yet another indication of how much antibiotics are overutilized worldwide.) The *E. coli* from the Boston kids had little resistance to any of eight different antibiotics, but the *E. coli* from children in China and Venezuela were already highly resistant.

Another study reported a high level of resistance to 75 percent of strains of gonococcus in countries with no restrictions on antibiotic use, but only 20 percent in countries with tight controls. And yet another study, from the University of Texas, demonstrated not only the greater prevalence of antibiotic-resistant bacteria in the Third World but how easily these bacteria can infiltrate the developed world. Students from the United States who were studying in Mexico returned with their intestinal bacteria carrying a resistance plasmid for the antibiotic trimethoprim, to which they had had no resistance before entering Mexico, and to which resistance in the United States in general was rare.

This sort of dangerous subtherapeutic (or nontherapeutic) dosing doesn't just originate on the street from Third World hucksters. Often when people in the developing countries take ill they are conditioned to go to a folk healer, such as the tribal medicine man in Africa or an "injection doctor" in southeast Asia, particularly in Laos. These healers traditionally use herbs and other non-Western remedies, but those have begun to fall out of favor. The belief that Western medicines are imbued with certain magical therapeutic and prophylactic powers has been growing in several developing countries for some time. Therefore, in an attempt to attract more patients to their dwindling practices, many traditional healers have begun to incorporate the techniques of Western marketing and give their patients what they want. They have introduced Western drugs such as antibiotics into their therapies. While presumably they are better intentioned than the street hawkers, the results are frequently the same. These practitioners of folk medicine have little or no training in the proper use of ethical pharmaceuticals, and the antibiotics they prescribe are almost always either subtherapeutic doses or given to treat diseases that don't require an antibiotic at all.

Even where some controls seemingly exist and a more competent performance would be expected, the situation is really no better. Mostly because of the shortage of physicians in the developing world, the legal role of prescribing and dispensing of drugs, including antibiotics, has fallen to the pharmacies. Whereas in the developed world, there is about 1 physician for every 520 people, this number is about 1 to 2,700 in most of the developing world, and in some cases the ratio of physicians to population may be as low as 1 to 17,000. But the pharmacies have the same casual attitude toward the dispensing of potentially dangerous drugs as the street vendors do.

I remember a personal experience with this. While visiting Rio de Janeiro on holiday in 1983, I came down with a sore throat and a low-grade fever. I wasn't concerned that I had a strep throat, only a viral cold. Since I had found that (contrary to what many of my colleagues believed) increased vitamin C intake and zinc lozenges almost always worked to abate my symptoms, I went from my hotel across the street to a large pharmacy. Fortunately the pharmacist understood some English. When I explained what I wanted, he quickly obliged me with the vitamin C. Although he didn't have the zinc lozenges, he offered me what he undoubtedly considered a superior substitute: ampicillin, neatly packaged in plastic bags of five capsules. He was not catering to me in this fashion because I was a physician—he never found that out. I quickly got the idea that he tried to sell ampicillin, or some other antibiotic, to customers who came into his shop for a variety of complaints. To my knowledge, this practice continues today.

Dr. Diana Melrose, of Oxfam in Britain, who has studied the problems of pharmaceutical abuse in Third World countries, relates a similar experience she had in North Yemen, where a supposedly trained pharmacist glibly recommended a very short course of a drug called Rivomycin Strepto, which he would have gladly provided, for her diarrhea.

A formal study of pharmaceutical dispensing in the developing world was conducted in Thailand a few years ago by Visanu Thamlikitkul from the division of infectious diseases at Siriraj Hospital in Bangkok. There was some attempt at supervision of the pharmacies, but as this study showed, it was meaningless. The drugstores in Thailand are divided into first-class and second-class stores. The first-class stores, of which there are about 1,800 in Bangkok, are required to have a registered pharmacist on duty at all times. He or she is the only one legally authorized to dispense antimicrobial agents without a prescription.

Forty fourth-year medical students were recruited to simulate patients in this study. They were instructed to fan out, each to a separate first-class drugstore, and present to the pharmacist a wide range of complaints, either for themselves or their children. The complaints included penile discharge, a wound in a four-year-old child, watery diarrhea in a six-month-old baby, fever with sore throat in both children and adults, and runny nose and cough in a two-month-old baby.

The results were nothing short of astonishing. The medical students might as well have consulted with a street vendor as with these Thai pharmacists. Only four of them refused to dispense medication to the two-month-old baby, and only one refused the six-month-old. In every other case, antibiotics were freely prescribed. Both the types of antibiotics and the dosage schedules varied widely, with no apparent rhyme or reason. And to further complicate matters, in no instance was a full course of the drug supplied. What was given ranged from a single dose to multiple doses lasting less than four days, with an average of two days. Even if the conditions had actually existed, all the doses would have been subtherapeutic and would have selected for resistant strains of bacteria.

Besides a general lack of education in the Third World on what antibiotics are for, poverty is another reason for their misuse that physicians and competent pharmacists are forced to deal with. Many people simply can't afford to take an entire course of antibiotics. Workers in the Dominican Republic and other countries often have to spend an entire day's wages on one day's worth of drugs. Taking medication for ten days would mean their families wouldn't eat. The choice for them is clear. The economics of the developing world undoubtedly corresponds to the packaging policies of the pharmacies. If they sell antibiotics only in a ten-day supply, they will sell none. From the proprietor's point of view, it's better to ring up a few capsules on the cash register than none.

Poverty, not surprisingly, creates still other problems. In the United States, Europe and Japan, if resistance to a drug such as penicillin or tetracycline develops, there are newer drugs available which may be better simply because they haven't been on the market as long and as a result resistance to them will be less prevalent. But these newer drugs are always more expensive. The governments of most Third World countries can't afford to import them. Therefore, there is a vicious cycle: because of lack of controls and previous abuses, the bacteria that cause diseases in the Third World are largely resistant to the only available drugs. Yet these drugs are administered. As a consequence, resistance becomes more and more entrenched, going to more and different plasmids and then eventually back to the developed world.

Third World physicians might be tempted to try another solution, such as pressuring their governments to enact more controls or to try to purchase at least limited supplies of newer antibiotics, if they weren't constantly being pulled in the opposite direction by the horde of pharmaceutical sales representatives on whom they rely for information about drug protocol. Even physicians in the industrialized world have difficulty keeping up with the latest developments in pharmaceuticals and tend to trust detail men. While there are strict regulations to adhere to and potentially stiff penalties to pay for violations in the United States, there is no Food and Drug Administration or comparable organization in most Third World countries. The pharmaceutical companies there can say pretty much whatever they want about a drug. And they do.

This situation has improved quite a bit in the past several years, however. Under pressure from research by Dr. Phillip R. Lee and Dr. Milton Silverman of the University of California, San Francisco (Dr. Lee is now assistant secretary of Health and Human Services in the Clinton administration), who first uncovered many of the unethical marketing practices as long ago as the 1970s, the International Federation of Pharmaceutical Manufacturers' Associations (IFPMA) promulgated a Code of Pharmaceutical Marketing Practices in 1981. Member companies were called upon to conduct all their dealings with "complete candor" and to restrict their claims to those that could be supported by scientific fact. According to follow-up research by Dr. Lee in the late 1980s, most of the large multinational member companies have been very good about complying with these regulations.

The IFMPA Code has been supplemented by legal action and dissemination of literature by several consumer groups. These include Health Action International (HAI), an umbrella for many consumer organizations worldwide; the International Organization of Consumer Unions (IOCU); Social Audit in England; and the recently formed Medical Lobby for Appropriate Marketing. The result of action by all of these groups has been the removal from the market of several ineffective or potentially harmful drugs, especially the dangerous or irrational combinations that are so common in the Third World. There has also been modification of several misleading advertising claims. Unfortunately, the ending is not entirely happy. Discrepancies still exist, because many of the smaller pharmaceutical firms, based in the Third World, have continued their unethical marketing, so physicians are still prescribing antibiotics for the wrong conditions—and the problem continues with no foreseeable end.

How much damage does the deplorable state of antibiotic use in the Third World actually do? It's been known to be a serious problem ever since 1969, when a dramatic pandemic of dysentery began in Guatemala and eventually spread to involve six Central American countries and southern Mexico before subsiding the following year. As many as 500,000 cases occurred during this epidemic, with many thousands of deaths. Much of the devastation was traced to an epidemic strain carrying an R-plasmid which imbued it with resistance to sulfa drugs, streptomycin, tetracycline and chloramphenicol.

A short time later, in 1972, a large outbreak of more than 10,000 cases of typhoid fever occurred in and around Mexico City. Later, in the 1970s and the 1980s, similar outbreaks of disease-carrying multiple antibiotic resistance surfaced in developing countries all over the world, from Mexico to Bangladesh, India, Burma, Sri Lanka and Zaire.

Also in the 1970s, a devastating cholera pandemic in Africa was caused by the so-called El Tor bacterium (a strain of *Vibrio cholerae*, the causative agent of cholera). Today in much of Africa, over 50 percent of these bacteria are resistant to tetracycline. Despite this widespread resistance, tetracycline continues to be used in almost astonishing amounts. Nothing has changed since Dr. Stuart Levy of Tufts University, a worldwide expert on antibiotic abuse, witnessed the following incident in 1981 while visiting a laboratory in Jakarta, Indonesia.

One hundred thousand Indonesian Muslims were to make a pilgrimage to Saudi Arabia, fulfilling a lifelong dream. The Indonesian Ministry of Religion was concerned, however, about the spread of disease among people traveling so far and for so long in such close quarters. The most likely disease they might contract was cholera. As a precaution, besides performing bacterial cultures on all foods served on the airplanes and trains, every one of the 100,000 pilgrims was given a course of tetracycline. Not only were these prophylactic doses ill advised in general, but with the bacteria already resistant to tetracycline, the administration of the antibiotic only worsened the problem. But this was the only drug the government had available. And this was the only way it could think of to combat the danger.

Not long after the epidemics went roaring full-force through the developing world, it was discovered that the resistance genes were not going to be confined. In many cases, travelers to these countries either came down with the same diseases—resistant to multiple antibiotics—or else became carriers of the antibiotic-resistance plasmids and brought them home.

We have also seen this same phenomenon of transfer of antibiotic resistance originate from instances that weren't catastrophic, or even noticed at the time, but which have caused us problems nonetheless. Until American servicemen went to Vietnam, gonorrhea in the Western world was universally sensitive to penicillin. But when Americans began to regularly frequent the brothels of Saigon, they acquired an unusual strain of gonorrhea that was almost completely resistant. The prostitutes in these brothels had, for some time, been receiving regular doses of penicillin to keep them free of disease. This perhaps well-intentioned but poorly advised practice had exactly the opposite effect. It eventually selected for the rare penicillin-resistant strains of gonococcus, which were transmitted to the American soldiers, who then brought them back to the United States. Today, it is rare to find a strain of gonococcus that is sensitive to penicillin anywhere in America or Europe.

And now that we are in the post–Cold War era, we can expect the exportation of antibiotic-resistant strains from places such as Hungary (where more than 50 percent of the pnemococci are already resistant to penicillin) and other countries that large numbers of Americans are traveling to for the first time. The situation doesn't have to be this way. A survey of antibiotic use in primary care clinics in Harare, Zimbabwe, demonstrated that it was possible to train the ancillary staff to prescribe antibiotics appropriately. The performance of these clinics was as good as that in most in the United States. And recently, in both Nigeria and Costa Rica, groups have begun speaking out and lobbying those responsible for health policy and purchasing to eschew the outmoded, dangerous antibiotics in favor of discreet use of the more effective ones. Of course, if the newer drugs are not used judiciously, the cycle will start all over again.

CHAPTER 7

Bigger Animals, More Resistance

A few years ago, I attended a scientific meeting at the University of California in Berkeley. At a Saturday evening social event, a dinner dance aboard a chartered ship, my wife and I were introduced to Dr. Thomas Jukes. I had known Dr. Jukes, now nearing the age of eighty-five and a professor emeritus of biology at Berkeley, to be a nutritional researcher of some prominence. He had done some of the seminal work on vitamin B_{12} in the 1940s and 1950s. But I was about to discover another aspect of Thomas Jukes. I was in the presence of the man whose work was arguably responsible for more antibiotic use in the United States than any other individual's.

In 1948, when Dr. Jukes was a young researcher at Lederle Laboratories, he and his colleague Robert Stokstad were looking for ways to improve growth in chickens. They were specifically hunting for sources of vitamin B_{12} that could be added to poultry feeds, most of which were prepared from soybean meal and were devoid of vitamin B_{12}, which is not produced by plants. A number of chance circumstances led them not only to what they were seeking but far beyond.

Only one year earlier at Lederle, another scientist, Benjamin Duggar, had isolated chlortetracycline (also known then as Aureomycin), the first of the tetracycline antibiotics, from soil bacteria. This had been hailed as a major breakthrough, and large-scale production of chlortetracycline was begun, employing huge vats of the soil bacteria. Once the antibiotic had been extracted, the vats remained filled with a mash of leftover bacteria, something for which Lederle had no other use, so Jukes and Stokstad claimed it, knowing that bacteria can produce vitamin B_{12}. Here, they thought, tailor-made for their purposes, was a cheap and readily available source of the vitamin.

When Jukes and Stokstad added the mash to the diet of young chicks, the growth that resulted was far greater than they could have expected. After only twenty-five days, the chicks eating the mash were almost *three times* the size of other chicks that had been given a purified source of vitamin B_{12} in their food. The scientists could hardly believe their eyes. This sort of growth was unheard of; it had to be something more than the effect of the B_{12}. To be certain their discovery wasn't an anomaly, Jukes and Stokstad repeated the experiment over and over, varying the conditions in every way they could think of. "Very few experiments have been repeated so many times," Dr. Jukes told me. And each time they saw a remarkable growth effect from the bacterial mash, although not always as dramatic as in their original experiment. Thoroughly excited by their finding, they dubbed their as yet unidentified compound a new nutritional "growth factor."

That growth factor turned out to be traces of the antibiotic chlortetracycline left in the fermentation tanks after extraction. And it was later discovered that tetracycline was not only a powerful growth stimulant in young chicks, it was equally effective in cattle and hogs.

When Jukes announced these findings at the American Chemical Society annual meeting in Philadelphia in 1950, they were widely trumpeted by the press. The *Daily Telegraph* in London headlined its story "Drug Speeds Growth Fifty Percent; Effect on Animals," and said that "the American Chemical Society has announced in Philadelphia that the drug Aureomycin, hitherto known for its anti-infection properties, is also one of the greatest growth-promoting substances ever discovered." In a very short time, this discovery became the biggest boon ever to livestock and poultry production, transforming it from the small business it still was in the early 1950s into the multibillion-dollar industry it is today.

Since Jukes had found that only minute amounts of tetracycline, about five parts per million, was just as powerful a growth stimulant as larger amounts, the additional cost to farmers and ranchers would be minimal. And since governmental regulatory agencies viewed the addition of the antibiotic to animal feed as a nutritional supplement rather than a therapeutic intervention, the antibiotics could be sold without a prescription. In fact, so unanimous was the approval for using the antibiotic in animal feed that the farmers weren't even given the option to use it or not. Frequently the antibiotic was added to the feed during manufacture, right along with vitamins and minerals.

When Jukes tried to duplicate the growth-stimulant effect with the only other available antibiotic, penicillin, he succeeded with it as well. Since that time, other antibiotics have been shown to have a growth-stimulant effect, but tetracycline and penicillin remain the most commonly used in animal feed.

Here's the rub. Antibiotics have been used for growth promotion for more than forty years, and we still don't know how they work to accomplish this result. Dr. Jukes told me he believes that all so-called normal young animals are marginally sick, that is, infected with bacteria. These bacteria, he explained, could slow growth in one of two ways, or a combination of both. They could compete directly with the animal for the limited supply of nutrients, or they could compete for nutrients with the friendly intestinal bacteria which make certain other nutrients (such as vitamin B_{12}). In either case, the antibiotics would make more nutrients available to the animal and speed growth. Although some other researchers have at times attributed some hidden, still undiscovered nutritional value to antibiotics, Dr. Jukes disputes this. Animals raised in a laboratory under strictly sterile conditions, in what is called a germ-free environment, do not benefit from the addition of antibiotics to their feed. They grow no faster. This implies that the effect of antibiotics is an antibacterial one. And antibiotics given to animals pass through their intestines unchanged. If they were providing some nutritional benefit, it would be logical to expect them to be somehow metabolized.

Why, after all this time, haven't the mystery bacteria responsible for making the animals sick been identified? Jukes's answer is that the intestine of a warm-blooded vertebrate contains some twenty-one trillion bacteria, many species of which still haven't been isolated.

When first introduced, the antibiotics provided a whole variety of benefits. Although sanitary conditions on many farms and feedlots are not ideal today, they were much worse forty years ago. Before the use of antibiotics, the land on which animals were raised was often contaminated by parasites that caused diseases. Bloody diarrhea caused death in young pigs, and chickens died by the thousands, suffocated by air-sac diseases. Baby calves frequently perished from a condition called scours. These problems were alleviated by antibiotics.

But it was the growth factor, unquestionably, that secured the use of antibiotics as routine. There are approximately six billion animals raised each year in the United States for human consumption, primarily cattle, swine and poultry, thirty times more than all the people in the United States, and more even than the total population of the world. Most of these animals receive antibiotics every day in their feed, from the time they are weaned until the day they are slaughtered. This amounts to about twenty million pounds of antibiotics a year, twice as much as is used in humans—although in the early days, the practice of using these drugs in this way almost spilled over into the human population. So successful were the animal results that Dr. Jukes and others began to experiment with and subsequently advocate the routine feeding of antibiotics to children, presumably believing that all young children were as marginally "sick" as young cattle. Even after all these years, Dr. Jukes says he still thinks it's a good idea and that if there were the same economic motivation to see children grow as fast as animals, it undoubtedly would be acted upon.

Not surprisingly, a huge problem developed. What was a boon to the meat and poultry industries turned out to be a bane to the health of the world.

Administering a subtherapeutic dose of an antibiotic to an animal can select for resistant strains of bacteria, in exactly the same way it does in people. The small amounts of antibiotics given to animals for growth promotion remain subtherapeutic doses even though they are given for long periods of time; the problem is only compounded by the repetition of the dose. If a microbiologist were designing a laboratory experiment under the most carefully controlled conditions, the purpose of which was to select for the greatest number of antibiotic-resistant bacteria, he couldn't come up with a better scheme than the one carried out on animals every day.

The resistant bacteria that result from this reckless practice do not stay confined to the animals in which they develop. There are no "cow bacteria" or "pig bacteria" or "chicken bacteria." In terms of the microbiological world, we humans along with the rest of the animal kingdom are all part of one giant ecosystem. The same resistant bacteria that grow in the intestinal tract of a cow or pig can, and do, eventually end up in our bodies.

In 1965, there was a large outbreak in England of food poisoning and diarrhea associated with *Salmonella*. Infections of this sort due to *Salmonella* are usually mild, and when they are severe enough to require antibiotic therapy, the response is generally rapid. In this case, however, many of the bacteria were resistant to several antibiotics, a situation that resulted in six human deaths. This epidemic occurred concomitantly with a rash of *Salmonella* cases in calves; and investigation revealed that almost 25 percent of the human *Salmonella* strains showed the same antibiotic-resistance pattern—to tetracycline as well as other antibiotics—as was found in the calves' *Salmonella*.

The seriousness of the outbreak led to an intensive inquiry by a group of government-appointed microbiologists and physicians called the Swann Committee. In 1969, the Swann Committee issued a report which concluded that subtherapeutic use of antibiotics in animals for long periods of time produces a strong selection for resistant bacteria in the intestinal flora of the animals and that these bacteria have a potential human risk. The committee recommended banning the routine use in animals of any antibiotic that was commonly used in human therapy. It also recommended that the use of antibiotics as a feed supplement should require a prescription written by a veterinarian. The recommendations were accepted in 1970, and since then the only antibiotics legally allowed to be used in Britain for growth promotion in animals are those prescribed by a veterinarian and not used in human medicine. This practice was soon adopted by several other European countries, including the Netherlands, all of Scandinavia, and Germany. It was adopted by Canada as well.

Soon after the ban was put into effect in these countries, the feeling that the same thing should be done in the United States was widely expressed. In April 1977, the Food and Drug Administration proposed to remove penicillin and tetracyclines from animal feed and place them solely on veterinary prescription "for the shortest time necessary to achieve the desired result." "The theoretical possibility that drug-resistant pathogens can be produced by antibiotic selection has become a real threat. . . ," the FDA said. "The point is that known routes of transfer exist by which antibiotic use in animals contributes to such threats."

Congress, however, never approved this ban on antibiotics. Whether or not there was behind-the-scenes lobbying by the livestock industry, the result was a request for more evidence linking antibiotic-resistant bacteria that cause human disease with the use of penicillin and tetracyclines for growth promotion.

Even before 1977, in fact even before Britain enacted legislation in 1970, the scientific community was sharply polarized on what action should be taken. And although much of the evidence the FDA requested in 1977 had already been provided, there was still disagreement. That disagreement continues.

Not surprisingly, Dr. Jukes is still solidly on the side of the benefits of feeding antibiotics to animals, and he summarized for me the beliefs of several influential scientists who share his point of view. According to him, the positive effect on growth has been observed for as much as thirty years at places such as Washington State University, The American Cyanamid Corporation (Lederle) and the University of Wisconsin. This growth promotion, he said, has continued despite the development of antibiotic resistance by the animals. According to him, there was no indication even now that disease had increased in the animals as a result of the resistant strains.

The various effects on animals notwithstanding, the crux of the issue, of course, is the effect of these antibiotics on human health. This is where the real controversy comes in. Dr. Jukes and several other scientists believe that there has not been conclusive evidence showing a definite link between antibiotic-resistant bacteria that cause human disease and the use of penicillin and tetracyclines for growth promotion in animals. The term "conclusive" is the catch. We are dealing here with a problem for which it may be impossible to offer definitive proof.

The same antibiotics are used to treat both animals and humans, so it's difficult to sort out which type of usage selects for what type of resistance. Dr. Calvin Kunin, chief of infectious disease at Ohio State University School of Medicine, believes that it is the overuse by physicians on humans and not the subtherapeutic use on animals that is the problem. He points out that resistance to the newest antibiotics—the third-generation cephalosporins and the fluoro-quinolones, for example—occurs because of inappropriate use on humans and has nothing to do with animals.

Whatever one believes, it is clear that there are no easy solutions to the problem. In December 1984, Vice President (then Congressman) Gore presided over a congressional subcommittee hearing on antibiotic resistance. The entire first day was devoted to the animal issue. One of the witnesses, Dr. Leon Sabath, a professor of medicine and infectious disease expert at the University of Minnesota, pointed out that there are four separate segments of antibiotic use, all of which contribute to the selection and propagation of resistant strains of bacteria: the subtherapeutic use for growth promotion in animals, therapeutic use in treating disease in animals, prophylactic use in humans, and disease treatment in humans. Limiting just one segment, he testified, wouldn't solve the problem. If we stopped using all antibiotics for growth promotion in animals, we would still have to contend with the inappropriate use in the medical community, and veterinarians would still have the freedom to prescribe antibiotics whenever they deemed fit. He pointed out that since the legislative ban on subtherapeutic antibiotic use in Britain in 1970, neither resistance nor antibiotic use has decreased at all. Most believe the reason is that farmers, unwilling to have to deal with longer growth periods and increased feeding costs, simply have asked veterinarians for antibiotic prescriptions, and apparently the veterinarians have complied. Dr. Sabath felt that since it had been established in the United Kingdom that a legislative ban on the subtherapeutic use of antibiotics wouldn't decrease total antibiotic use at all, it was fruitless to consider it.

Humans can pick up the genes of resistant bacteria from animals in a variety of ways. The most direct way is through eating meat, especially undercooked or raw. As to more indirect gene transfers, Dr. Stuart Levy of Tufts University School of Medicine, one of the foremost researchers in the world on antibiotic abuse, has estimated that a cow will excrete about one hundred times the fecal matter of a human every day. Resistant bacteria that are produced in the intestinal tract of the cow will be excreted in the fecal matter, and most of them have the ability to survive. Often this same fecal material is used to fertilize produce, either directly or after treatment to form a slurry. In either case, the resistant bacteria are added to the soil and are incorporated by the vegetables and fruits as they grow.

There has been an increasing concern in recent years over pesticide residue on produce, but at least there is evidence that these toxic materials can be washed off in the kitchen if the proper solvents are used. In contrast, resistant bacteria and antibiotic-resistance genes persist even after washing. In fact washing, by pushing bacteria deep into existing crevices, can make things even worse. This means that vegetarians—even those who eat only organically grown produce—may not be protected from exposure to antibiotic-resistance genes.

Even when animal excrement isn't used as fertilizer, the resistant bacteria have other ways of spreading around the environment, especially via contact with birds, insects (flies are particularly adept at transporting bacteria long distances) and other animals which eventually bring the resistant bacteria to us.

Farmworkers, in particular, are vulnerable to picking up antibiotic-resistance genes from animals. No matter how careful one is, bacteria are ubiquitous. They can be swallowed or enter through the nose or even through the skin. More than fifteen years ago, Dr. Stuart Levy's laboratory group at Tufts University Medical School examined what happens when subtherapeutic levels of tetracycline, the same amounts that were normally used for growth promotion, were introduced into a farm environment. They divided three hundred newly hatched chicks into six different cages. Four cages were kept inside a barn and two were placed outside. Half the chicks received feed containing tetracycline; the other half didn't. Over the next nine months, the researchers examined the feces of all the chicks as well as the farmworkers and their families.

They discovered that within less than two days after beginning the feeding, the majority of the E. coli bacteria in the intestines of the chicks given tetracycline were resistant to the antibiotic, and over the next three months the bacteria developed resistance to ampicillin, as well as to streptomycin and sulfa drugs, even though none of the chicks, nor anyone on the farm, had been given those antibiotics at all.

Just as disturbing was that over a period of about six months, the same resistance pattern began to be seen in the farmworkers and their family members, beginning first with resistance to tetracycline and followed by resistance to the other antibiotics. It was well documented that none of these people took any antibiotics, including tetracycline, nor did they eat the chickens.

In a conversation I had with Dr. Kunin of Ohio State University, he dismissed as purely theoretical the concern that feeding one antibiotic to animals might subsequently lead to the development of resistance to multiple antibiotics and that this might then be transferred to humans. But Dr. Levy's study demonstrates that it is far more than a hypothesis.

And it is not the only study to show this forbidding prospect. In fact, studies conducted on pigs on farms in what was East Germany in the late 1980s carried the transfer of multiple-antibiotic-resistance genes even further. Within six months after introducing the antibiotic streptothricin into the pigs' feed for growth promotion, the resistance gene showed up in their intestinal bacteria. Two years later, the same resistance gene was recovered from the stools not only of many of the farmworkers but also of people who didn't even live on the farm but merely in the same area.

Although the bacteria acquired from the animals that carry these antibiotic-resistance genes aren't necessarily more likely to cause disease, once a disease is contracted multiple antibiotic resistance will make it very difficult to treat. In some cases it will be impossible.

Despite the inability of any American scientific body to suggest a legislative ban on the addition of antibiotics to animal feed, things are moving in that direction anyway. In the past few years, for example, the Cattlemen's Association has taken an unprecedented step and recommended that its members stop the routine use of common antibiotics as growth promoters and instead follow the British example, employing only those antibiotics not used in treatment of human disease. There is strong evidence that many livestock ranchers are heeding this advice and using instead a chemical called monensin. And other chemicals of this sort are becoming available. The poultry industry may be heading in the same direction, but the pork industry still uses tetracycline and penicillin.

Largely through organizations such as the National Resources Defense Council and Food Animal Concerns Trust (FACT), the public is being made more aware of the dangers, creating pressure where it is most felt—in the marketplace—and demanding animals raised without antibiotics. Consequently, we are beginning to see more of these products available. FACT, based in Chicago, has launched a chicken-egg product called Nest Eggs, produced by free-range chickens on farms in New Jersey and Illinois. These chickens are raised without any antibiotics added to their feed and are allowed to roam and scratch, instead of being crowded into tight cages as is common in the poultry industry. These same free-range chickens are becoming increasingly available in supermarkets and better restaurants. What was thought to be a fringe movement started by health fanatics has gained a solid head of scientific steam. If it keeps going, we will begin to see major changes in this area of antibiotic usage, a giant step in the direction of better health.

But even as we are developing some solutions to the livestock problem, we are facing continued and new challenges from other areas. Agribusiness is one example. Not only do antibiotics get into our fruits and vegetables via the fertilizer route, in some instances the drugs are applied directly to the plants. This practice is extremely common in fruit orchards. Just like people, plants are vulnerable to a variety of bacterial infections, and many growers apply the antibiotics in an attempt to prevent these diseases at particularly vulnerable points in the growing cycle. Although the antibiotics are occasionally injected directly into the tree trunks, more often they are sprayed, either by huge ground-based machines or from airplanes. While this may be a more efficient way of getting antibiotics into the trees, it also spreads them onto many other bystander plants. This leads to more bacterial resistance to antibiotics, which can then be transferred to humans. Even though the plant bacteria rarely cause disease in humans, the resistance genes are now residing in the intestinal tract and can eventually be donated to disease-causing bacteria.

The fish industry is another area where antibiotics are being used more and more. As we have become aware of the health benefits of eating fish, our consumption has increased, and fish farms are sprouting up around the United States, producing catfish, trout and salmon, imitating practices already in place for many years in Japan and Scandinavia, where the majority of fish consumed are cultured rather than caught. In whatever country it takes place, most of these fish are given antibiotics in their feed. There is little evidence that a growth-promoting effect exists for fish as for other animals, but many species are susceptible to bacterial diseases, so antibiotics are used frequently. By law in the United States, the administration of the drugs must be stopped several weeks before the fish are sold for consumption. This ensures that there will be no antibiotic residue in the fish (for which they are periodically inspected), but it does not protect against the presence of antibiotic-resistant bacteria (for which the fish are not inspected).

In addition, antibiotics are indiscriminately given to our pets, either by small-animal veterinarians or sometimes by the pet owners themselves. In virtually all pet stores, there are antibiotics for sale without prescription. These are meant mostly for fish hobbyists, but there are numerous accounts of the same antibiotics being given to dogs and cats, and even sometimes taken by the pet owners themselves. This is not a trivial matter. There are more than 150 million cats and dogs in the United States alone, as well as countless fish and birds as pets. The indiscriminate administration of antibiotics to them can account for a significant increase in the global pool of resistant bacteria. Thus it is imperative that we address each of these areas of antibiotic abuse as diligently as we have begun to address the livestock and poultry problem.

CHAPTER 8

First Cures, First Problems

Besides being a gifted scientist, Alexander Fleming was also a typically stoic Scotsman. Hence it is rare in any of his writings, even his diaries or letters, to find interjections of personal feelings. Still, he must have felt a sharp stab of disappointment in 1941 when word reached him that penicillin, the antibiotic he had discovered in 1928, had failed its first clinical trial.

On December 27, 1940, a forty-three-year-old policeman had been admitted to the Radcliffe Infirmary in Oxford. One month earlier he had scratched his face on a rosebush, a superficial scratch he thought nothing of at the time. But this commonplace incident quickly turned into something extraordinary. Instead of promptly healing, the cut became infected with an aggressive *Staphylococcus*. Within a few weeks the bacteria spread from his skin into the deeper tissues of his face and scalp, producing multiple abscesses which, despite the administration of massive doses of sulfa drugs—the only antibacterial agent then available—became so severe that in early February one eye had to be removed. By then, however, the bacteria had reached his lungs, and at the time of his admission to the infirmary he was near death, with a racking cough, a temperature approaching 105 degrees, shaking chills and severe lethargy.

The admitting physicians held little hope of saving him, but there was one last chance. Only a few months earlier, two Oxford physicians, Howard Florey and Ernst B. Chain, had succeeded in partially purifying crude extracts of penicillin and believed they had learned how to produce it in quantities that might be able to be used clinically. The potential of their accomplishment had excited certain members of the medical community, but Florey and Chain had yet to test their purified penicillin on even one human patient. And being careful scientists, they were reluctant to do so, under such uncontrolled conditions, when they were approached by the dying patient's doctors for some of the perhaps lifesaving antibiotic. They had no idea what might happen. But the desperation of Dr. Charles Fletcher was so convincing that in the end they agreed to give him all the precious penicillin they had.

Physicians began to inject the partially purified drug intravenously into the dying policeman every three hours round the clock. After just two days, however, they ran out of penicillin. Florey and Chain had no more, nor did anyone else. The world's supply of purified extract had literally been depleted. But rather than give up, the doctors ingeniously collected their patient's urine, extracted the penicillin from it, and reinjected it into his veins. They were operating blind, not knowing at all if the urine extract would have any effect, therapeutic or toxic. Their diligence was rewarded, however. On the fifth day the policeman finally appeared to be coming out of his near coma. His temperature dropped to almost normal and his chills disappeared. He sat up in bed and took meals. The Radcliffe doctors and the policeman's family were elated but their joy was short-lived. Although the urine collections, extractions and reinjections continued, they abruptly stopped working. Within just a few days the fever and chills returned with a vengeance, the policeman began coughing up blood-tinged sputum, and while the doctors stood by helplessly, he died shortly thereafter of staphylococcal pneumonia.

Because this clinical trial had been an emergency, unplanned one, the parameters of which were not known, the unsuccessful results were kept rather quiet. Most of the world outside the tight-knit British microbiological community never heard that the first attempt at heroism with purified penicillin had failed. Apparently even in early 1941, before the life of one patient had been saved, it was felt that the potential for penicillin was too great for its public image to be tarnished.

But Alexander Fleming heard of it and knew just what it meant. The patient received round-the-clock intravenous doses of purified penicillin for five days—more than forty injections of the most concentrated material available—and yet the staphylococci were only partially subdued, able to mount a full-force attack once the supply of penicillin was exhausted. Fleming must have known why. Florey and Chain had been attempting to treat the first known case of a *Staphylococcus* that was resistant to penicillin. The early injections had been successful because the drug had killed off most of the bacteria that were susceptible to the penicillin. But the resistant strains remained and grew back when the antibiotic was stopped.

As disappointing as it was to see it demonstrated clinically, the existence of penicillin-resistant *Staphylococcus* couldn't have come as a great shock to Fleming, nor to Florey and Chain. Although he had not yet seen it in staphylococci, Fleming knew from his original experiments that there were some strains of bacteria that penicillin didn't inhibit. And it was Chain, along with another Oxford colleague, Edward Abraham, who earlier that year had written a letter to the editor of the journal *Nature* in which they described the existence of a bacterial enzyme able to inactivate penicillin. They named the enzyme penicillinase. But Abraham and Chain had not discovered this enzyme in *Staphylococcus* either. They had isolated it from *E. coli*, the same bacteria that Fleming had observed were unaffected by penicillin. Now, however, this treatment failure meant it was probable that this same penicillin-destroying enzyme existed in certain strains of *Staphylococcus*. Could this mean that penicillin wasn't quite the miracle drug everyone was hoping it would be?

In 1942, a team of doctors at the Johns Hopkins Hospital in Baltimore became aware of the fact that while the crude extract of penicillin (it was still two years until Florey and Chain's purified penicillin would be mass-produced) was quite capable of killing pneumococci, streptococci and staphylococci, certain strains of all these organisms showed resistance. In some of them, the resistance to penicillin was so great that the bacteria could actually flourish in nutrient broth that contained relatively high concentrations of the crude extract.

That same year in London, similar strains of resistant *Staphylococcus* were isolated, and Abraham and Chain demonstrated what had been suspected, that these bacteria were indeed capable of manufacturing penicillinase. Some of these resistant strains were isolated from patients at Fleming's own hospital, the venerable St. Mary's. Upon realizing this, Fleming felt compelled to issue a cautionary warning to physicians to be on guard for these resistant strains when treating patients and that incomplete treatments could foster the growth of these resistant bacteria. He repeated this warning to the general public in a 1945 interview that appeared in *The New York Times,* ironically at the same time he was touring the United States and receiving accolades for having discovered penicillin.

These resistant strains of staphylococci were easily spread from infected hospital patients to other patients, and many doctors and nurses became carriers. This phenomenon developed with amazing speed. By 1946, 12 percent of the staphylococci isolated from patients at Hammersmith Hospital in London were resistant to penicillin. In the next two years, the percentage of resistant strains rose to 38 and then to 59.

This naturally had an impact on the ability to treat diseases with penicillin. In 1945, penicillin treatment reduced fatalities caused by *Staphylococcus* to only one-fourth of patients infected, but by 1953 only about half could be saved, and just two years later, in 1955, an amazing 80 percent of patients infected with *Staphylococcus* died. Thus, in only fifteen short years after the first documented treatment failure with penicillin, the antibiotic was rendered virtually ineffective against the most dangerous organism of the day, and the one on which Fleming had made his monumental discovery.

But even as the chinks in penicillin's armor began to appear in the early 1940s, the drug was being hailed as a godsend. Most of the world, even most of the medical community, seemed unaware that penicillin might be somewhat less than perfect. The mood of optimism had been slowly building since 1928 and Fleming's celebrated discovery. And the story of how this happened has since become almost as famous as the antibiotic itself. Some of the minor details vary, depending on exactly which version one chooses to believe, but there is no doubt it was an extraordinary turn of events. If serendipity has been responsible for many great scientific discoveries, what happened to Alexander Fleming in September 1928 was the result of pure cosmic timing.

On either the third or fourth of September, 1928, Fleming returned to his laboratory at St. Mary's Hospital for what was to be a brief visit. He had been on holiday with his family at their country retreat in Suffolk and had been summoned back hastily by a colleague, who requested help in treating a patient with a recalcitrant abscess. Although not yet chairman of the famed inoculation department at St. Mary's, Fleming already enjoyed a reputation as a skilled diagnostician and bacteriologist and was the likely consultant for this problem. After helping out with the patient, Fleming stopped in at his laboratory to do a little work before returning to the country. He never did complete his holiday.

Fleming sat down at his workbench and began to sort through the pile of petri dishes (also called plates) containing agar and nutrient growth medium which he had left there. In one account, by David Masters in a biography of Fleming, he is said to have held one particular dish to the light. Upon recognizing something unusual, he turned to his laboratory colleague, Dr. E. W. Todd, and said, "Now look at this, this is very interesting. I like this sort of thing—it might be important."

But most biographies of Fleming, including the ones by Sir Ronald Hare, Professor Emeritus of Bacteriology at the University of London, and Gwynn MacFarlane, the eminent British physician and author, report a slightly different version of events. Although essentially similar to the first, it has become the more widely accepted story, probably at least in part because it is more dramatic.

In this variation, Fleming didn't find the famous petri dish on his workbench but rather discovered it sitting with several others in a tray of Lysol disinfectant, waiting to be discarded. Fortunately the gods were with him that day. The stack of petri dishes in the disinfectant was so tall that the plate in question was left high and dry. Had it been submerged in the disinfectant, what was on the plate would have been destroyed and the world would have had to wait for another time—and another scientist—for penicillin.

Sitting down at his bench, Fleming noticed how many plates he had left in the discard pile. This prompted him to complain to a colleague, who had dropped in to visit, about how much work he had to do. Contrary to what we might expect of a scientist of his stature, Fleming was not a workaholic. Although dedicated and meticulous, he generally worked only six hours a day, reserving time every late afternoon to play snooker with friends at his men's club before going home to dinner. To demonstrate how hard he had been working, he then picked up one of the plates off the top of the pile to show his colleague, noticed something unusual and said simply, "That's funny!"

Whatever he actually said, he was looking at hundreds of colonies of staphylococcal bacteria, exactly what he had inoculated on the plates and would have expected to be growing. It was one area of the plate, however, that he found unusual. There was a distinct colony of fungus growing, something he hadn't inoculated on the plate. And in the vicinity of the fungus, and only in that area, there was a dramatic reduction in the number of bacterial colonies. This area had a transparent, almost clear look that Fleming later referred to as "ghosts." Somehow the fungus was causing the colonies to lyse, or dissolve.

This phenomenon was of great interest to Fleming, but not (at least initially) for the reasons we might expect. Since 1922, Fleming had been occupied with refining the properties of a substance he had discovered in several body fluids. Because of its capacity to dissolve bacteria, he thought the compound was an enzyme and called it lysozyme. Never considered to have any potential use in clinical medicine, lysozyme could dissolve only non-disease-causing bacteria. Fleming's interest in the compound was purely intellectual, and he thought on that morning only that he had found another type of lysozyme, one produced by mold rather than by human body fluids. Even though this lysozyme was different in another way—it *had* affected staphylococci, disease-causing bacteria—Fleming still didn't think of it at the time as being of therapeutic importance. Yet, something told him that this was not just another piece of data to be recorded in a laboratory notebook. Having worked on lysozyme for some time, he undoubtedly had the "prepared mind" that Pasteur said nature favors. Fleming was known for possessing uniquely keen powers of observation and intuition, powers that extended even outside the scientific arena. He is said, for example, to have advised a colleague one afternoon in 1925 at a Sotheby's auction to gamble three pounds to acquire two paintings by a little-known artist named Pablo Picasso.

Eighteen years later, on February 20, 1946, in a lecture at the Mayo Clinic in the United States, Fleming revealed what his first impressions of penicillin had been. With the gift of hindsight, he described what had happened as follows:

"I need not go into details of the research on which I was engaged at the time but my culture plate was covered with staphylococcal colonies. The particular work involved opening the plate and looking at it under a dissecting microscope and then leaving it for growth to take place. That, of course, was asking for trouble by contamination, as things were always dropping from the air and sure enough, trouble came but led to penicillin. A mold spore, coming from I don't know where, dropped on the plate. That didn't excite me. I had seen such contamination before, but what I had never seen before was staphylococci undergoing lysis around the contaminating colony. Obviously something extraordinary was happening."

But according to Sir Ronald Hare, this chance discovery was far more bizarre than Fleming had either remembered or revealed to his audience at the Mayo Clinic or in any of his writings. His good fortune that the plate hadn't been disinfected was only one piece of the intricate puzzle. There were still several scientific facts that didn't quite fit Fleming's story. These inconsistencies apparently dogged Hare for decades until finally in the 1980s, well into his seventies, he was able to replicate the steps necessary for penicillin to be discovered in exactly the same way that Fleming had discovered it. What he accomplished was a piece of British detective work worthy of Scotland Yard.

Hare found it easy to inhibit the growth of new bacterial colonies. This is, after all, what we count on penicillin to do when it is used medically. But growth inhibition is not the same as lysis, the phenomenon that Fleming had observed. Sorting this out, Hare felt, was of great historical importance. Since lysis was what Fleming had been working on, had he seen growth inhibition—which would have looked significantly different—he might not have proceeded. Lysis involves the dissolving of already existing colonies; because penicillin's chief mode of action is to disrupt the synthesis of the bacterial cell wall, it normally can affect the organisms only when they are in the process of dividing, not once they are already formed. For lysis to occur, a variety of complex conditions has to coexist.

So how did Fleming come to observe lysis? The only way that could have happened, reasoned Hare, was that somehow the mold contaminated the petri dish at approximately the same time Fleming inoculated it with staphylococci. If either organism had preceded the other, lysis wouldn't have occurred. That was relatively easy to deduce. But what had to happen next? If Fleming had then put the petri dish in the incubator, as he would normally have done, the famous plate would have ended up in the autoclave to be recycled instead of in the archives of St. Mary's Hospital, where it remains today. This is because staphylococci, like most bacteria, grow very well at incubator temperatures (37 degrees centigrade, the same as normal body temperature). Most fungi, on the other hand, don't grow as well at that temperature. They do far better at room temperature. In the incubator, the staphylococci would have simply overgrown the plate and choked out the fungus. There would have been no subsequent lysis.

Therefore, Hare concluded that Fleming had originally left the plate at room temperature, on his workbench, and it had never made it into the incubator. But why would Fleming, a careful bacteriologist, have forgotten to put the plate into the incubator? It didn't at all fit with his compulsive demeanor. The answer lies in some other work he had been doing.

Early in 1928, Fleming had been asked by Britain's Medical Research Council to write a review on staphylococci. Although already considered an authority on the subject, in order to be as complete as possible, Fleming conducted an exhaustive search through the literature and came across a paper which had originated from the School of Pathology at Trinity College in Dublin. The report by Joseph Bigger and his colleagues described how colonies of *Staphylococcus* had the ability to take on unusual structures when incubated at various temperatures, including room temperature. It is quite likely that Fleming was trying to repeat Bigger's observations before he left on holiday in July, and therefore intentionally left the petri dish to grow at room temperature on his workbench.

Even London, however, experiences heat waves in the summer, and meteorological records for 1928 indicate that it was an unusually hot July. In those days before air conditioning a laboratory could become in effect an incubator and despite being left at room temperature, the bacteria, again, might have overwhelmed the mold. The reason why it did not lies in a more detailed examination of the weather patterns, and yet another extraordinary circumstance. Just after Fleming left for the country, the temperature turned from exceptionally warm to exceptionally cool, the perfect environment for growing the contaminating mold. Then, in August, another heat wave enveloped London, allowing the staphylococci to grow. It was virtually only this combination of meteorological occurrences that could have accounted for the growth of both the fungus and the bacteria in the proper sequence for subsequent lysis to occur.

Still another question Professor Hare needed to answer was from where the contaminating mold originated. Once again, several popular versions of Fleming's discovery ascribed a sloppy technique to him that wouldn't fit. Because of the unusually warm summer in London that year, it was said that Fleming had developed the habit of leaving the window open in his laboratory, thereby providing a ready entrance for the contaminating mold. But open windows are anathema to any self-respecting bacteriologist, let alone Fleming. "Fleming had devoted his life's work to the study of bacteria, and good sterile technique was second nature to him, so he would never have had the window open while inoculating the plates," writes Milton Wainwright in *Miracle Cure*, an account of Fleming and his discovery. In addition, the penicillin-producing mold that Fleming happened on was not a particularly common member of the spore population of nonlaboratory air. It almost certainly came from somewhere else.

That somewhere else turned out to be the laboratory just below Fleming's. It was occupied by a young physician, a mycologist (a specialist in fungi) named C. J. La Touche, who at that time was collecting fungi from all over London, in an attempt to prove they were involved in causing asthma. He too was a careful scientist, but it seems likely that despite all precautions some of his mold spores contaminated the air in his laboratory and were then carried upstairs to the laboratory where Fleming was working. Hare was even methodical enough to examine carefully the two rooms and determine it was the connecting shaft of a dumbwaiter running between the two laboratories that was the conduit that had brought the fungus to Fleming's lab.

As confirmation that the fungus came from Dr. La Touche's collection, several months after having determined that it was penicillin he had discovered and not another lysozyme, Fleming went to his scientific neighbor and asked for samples of all the molds he had. He wanted to see if penicillin production was a common characteristic of molds in general. None of La Touche's samples produced penicillin, however, except one, a culture that had exactly the same characteristics growing on a petri dish as Fleming's isolate. Had any other of La Touche's molds blown up the dumbwaiter shaft, there would have been no penicillin produced.

We have, then, an almost unbelievable constellation of circumstances and events that led to Fleming's discovery. The mold itself was a rare strain, one that the scientist in the laboratory immediately below him happened to be working on; it had to be that particular mold that went up the airshaft and contaminated Fleming's plate. Further, it was necessary that Fleming leave the petri dish at room temperature, rather than in the incubator; that there be several days of first cold and then hot weather; that the stack of discarded plates be piled so high in the disinfectant solution that the plate with the penicillin was left exposed; and that a visit from a laboratory colleague stimulate Fleming to look at the discarded plate on top. "Omit any of these factors and the discovery of penicillin might be postponed indefinitely!" concluded Dr. James G. Hirsch, the former dean of graduate studies at Rockefeller University in New York.

Having been the beneficiary of all of this, however, it was then left to Fleming to take advantage of his discovery. Had he not acted upon his observations, they would have led nowhere. He first attempted to repeat his initial observation of lysis. Not being aware of the circumstances that produced the effect, he of course was unable to do so. Nevertheless, rather than abandon it and continue with other, more immediately promising areas of his work, some inner gyroscope drove him to persist.

It was already well accepted by microbiologists in 1928 that certain organisms, bacteria and others, could inhibit growth of other microorganisms. This, however, was thought to be purely on a competitive basis, by one denying nutrients to the other, changing the acidity of the surrounding environment or otherwise making conditions unfavorable for growth. But Fleming, in another demonstration of his superior scientific mind, came to realize that, while he couldn't repeat lysis, this mold which had contaminated his petri dish of *Staphylococcus* was inhibiting the growth of the bacteria, and it must be doing so, not by competing with it for nutrients, but by excreting an antibacterial agent. He remarked in his writing that if this agent could be extracted and purified it might play an important role in the fight against infection.

Once he recognized that the fungus was producing an antibacterial agent, Fleming set about producing large quantities of what he called "mold juice" in order to be able to study the properties of the substance in greater detail and eventually to purify it. As physician and author Milton Wainwright has written, "If Fleming expected this last task to be straightforward, then he was disappointed. In fact, the purification step would always elude him."

Fleming, with the help of La Touche, identified the mold as *Penicillium notatum*. Following that, he chose the name penicillin for his compound. He then made the decision to publish his work and on May 10, 1929, some eight months after having first come upon the contaminated petri dish, submitted a paper to the *British Journal of Experimental Pathology*. It was promptly accepted and published the next month. The paper mainly summarized the results of Fleming's studies on penicillin, including the cultural conditions that promoted growth of the mold and encouraged it to produce penicillin. Fleming also wrote of another finding: that penicillin had a selective effect on bacteria, and it didn't inhibit all types. While it markedly suppressed the growth of staphylococci and the diphtheria bacillus, it didn't inhibit the bacteria that caused typhoid fever. He then described his unsuccessful attempts in the laboratory to purify penicillin and made the point that the crude extract was nonirritant to body tissue. And finally, and perhaps most important, he referred to the possible clinical usefulness of penicillin: "It is suggested that it may be an efficient antiseptic for application to, or injection into, areas affected by penicillin-sensitive microbes."

This statement, which seems so obvious today, was almost not included in the paper. Dr. Almoth Wright, the head of Fleming's department, didn't believe that penicillin might have any therapeutic value and strongly advised against any reference to that possibility. As V. D. Allison, Fleming's close friend, wrote in 1979, "Wright had been the reverse of enthusiastic about the curative value of penicillin when the manuscript of the first paper was submitted for publication. So much so that he had demanded the omission of the short paragraph suggesting its employment for surface infections—meaning local infections." Fleming, however, stood his ground, not an easy task considering that Wright was both internationally famous and an autocrat.

It was also difficult because of the prevailing mood of the day. Although not all bacteriologists believed, as did Almoth Wright, that penicillin wouldn't be effective even on superficial infections, the notion that intravenous therapy, the injecting of some antibacterial compound into the body, would be effective in treating infections was widely discredited.

Almost as if determined to prove his boss wrong, immediately after his research paper had been accepted, Fleming set out to demonstrate the antibacterial effectiveness of penicillin. Working with crude extracts of the fungus, he and a colleague began to use it on superficial infections such as boils and leg ulcers, with moderate success at best. In fact, the only definitive cure Fleming ever achieved with penicillin was when he applied the remarkably foul-smelling broth to the eye of his laboratory assistant and completely cleared up a superficial infection.

In retrospect, even this minor achievement was somewhat of a miracle. The crude fungal extracts contained almost no penicillin at all, and it rather quickly became clear that if penicillin were to have any significant therapeutic effect, it would have to be purified and concentrated. Whether Fleming actually tried to accomplish this isn't known, but he didn't succeed, most probably because his knowledge of biochemistry—needed in order to extract the penicillin from the fungus—was rudimentary at best.

It took another decade before anyone succeeded. Aware of his biochemical shortcomings, Fleming passed the mantle to several former students. One of them, Lewis Holt, had a doctorate in biochemistry and in 1934 actually performed a crucial step necessary for purification. But he never realized the significance of what he had done, and thus missed his chance to share immortality with Fleming.

Holt's failure was really Fleming's, and St. Mary's Hospital's, last direct work with penicillin. Fleming was clearly discouraged at the inability to purify penicillin, but even so remained optimistic about its potential. In 1934 he told another doctor at St. Mary's that penicillin might prove beneficial in the treatment of venereal disease. The doctor, G. L. M. McElligot, described their discussion to Milton Wainwright as follows: "I shall not forget the day in 1934 when he showed me the famous contaminated culture with the prophetic comment, 'That stuff should be good for your patients,' and how the subsequent discussion on ways and means ended with his saying, 'It's up to the chemists now. I'm no chemist.' "

For the next few years, the scene shifted briefly to the United States, where a few prominent physicians attempted to use penicillin on patients, and several of the major pharmaceutical companies—mainly Merck, but also Squibb, Lederle, Lilly and Parke Davis—showed an interest in purifying it, but never succeeded. Until 1938, penicillin remained for many a laboratory curiosity.

It was then, at Oxford, that Florey and Chain began their momentous work, resulting in an accomplishment that in terms of its importance to medicine parallels Fleming's discovery. Fleming's name, however, is known to most of us; few outside the scientific community have ever heard of Howard Florey and Ernst Chain. Lest we assume that Fleming took the limelight for himself at the expense of his contemporaries, it was Florey and Chain who deliberately chose to stay well out of the public eye. Fleming, already sixty years old and nearing the end of his career, was happy to accept the accolades others shunned.

Florey had recently become interested, not in penicillin per se, but in lysozyme, the earlier of Fleming's discoveries, and had put his student Chain to work on it. Once he had finished the assigned project, Florey suggested that Chain might wish to look at some other antibacterial agents. And after reading through more than two hundred papers on microbial antagonism, Chain was drawn to Fleming's famous paper. Florey, who had been on the editorial board of the *British Journal of Experimental Pathology* nine years earlier when Fleming's manuscript was accepted, encouraged this research.

But neither Florey nor Chain was motivated by anything other than basic scientific interest. As of 1938, the only cures with crude penicillin had been the minor ones achieved by Fleming and a few others by students of his. Chain admitted that he had virtually no idea he might be working on a lifesaving drug and that had he been working at a pharmaceutical house rather than in an academic environment, it is very unlikely he would have obtained permission to do any research on penicillin.

Chain's first task was to get some penicillin—it was still a rare commodity. But in yet another of the amazing coincidences surrounding the penicillin story, there was someone already working with it in the pathology department at Oxford, not for any therapeutic research, but rather using it to separate bacteria.

Although the work went slowly at first, eventually Florey and Chain recognized that penicillin was not an enzyme or protein as Fleming had assumed, but a small molecule. This took them along the correct chemical path that within a year led to the first purified penicillin. Actually, it was only semi-pure, a yellow compound the British press called "Yellow Magic." The later, far more purified compound, similar to what we use today, was pure white.

Following toxicity studies, penicillin began its first major tests in animals just as Britain was entering World War II. Florey and Chain's associate, Norman Heatley, performed the experiments. Heatley injected eight mice with a highly virulent strain of streptococci; to four of them, he also gave the purified penicillin extract. Heatley remained in the lab until almost four o'clock in the morning, when the four control animals were dead. The treated animals seemed well. When he returned at noon the next day, the animals given penicillin were still perfectly well. The scientists could hardly contain their pleasure.

These results were published in August 1940, in the *Lancet*, but rather than causing a huge stir in the pharmaceutical industry, inexplicably they were virtually ignored. Fleming, however, was excited by this paper and made the journey unannounced from London to Oxford on September 2, 1940, almost twelve years to the day after he had discovered penicillin. Fleming and Florey got along quite well for some time, exchanging samples and ideas. Florey's lab was transformed into a penicillin-production factory, which hired young workers he called "penicillin girls" to inoculate flasks and later extract the penicillin.

Then came the penicillin failure with the case of the Oxford policeman, but soon after there was a case that provided a stage for penicillin to perform its first miracle. A young boy was admitted into the Oxford Infirmary with a particularly bad case of osteomyelitis in his left femur, caused by a staphylococcus. The first treatment, as it was for practically all infections those days, was sulfa drugs. When it was unsuccessful, doctors gave the boy penicillin intravenously. Just as with the policeman, if it proved ineffective, the boy would surely die, but within a few days he was feeling better. Although penicillin was being produced as rapidly as possible by Florey, the supply was still quickly exhausted, and the doctors followed the same procedure as before, using the patient's urine as a secondary source. This time, however, the miracle wasn't temporary; there was no relapse. Penicillin had saved the boy from certain death. And in London, Fleming must have allowed himself a smile, which lasted at least until some of the bad reviews came rolling in.

With this success, things moved with alacrity from laboratory to clinic. But it was the Americans, not the British, who were the first to produce penicillin on a mass scale. Although Florey approached British pharmaceutical companies, the drug industry was too disrupted by the constant bombing of the war to develop any sort of coherent program. But with the help of the U.S. government, several American firms and scientists, penicillin began rolling off the production lines by 1944. Robert Coghill, head of the fermentation division at the Northern Regional Research Laboratory in Peoria, Illinois (a division of the U.S. Department of Agriculture), recalls his feeling on a winter morning in 1944, when he visited Pfizer's production plant in Brooklyn and stood before the huge fermentation tanks, each of which was capable of producing ten thousand gallons of crude broth containing penicillin. "I stood at the end of the production line and saw one-hundred-thousand-unit vials of penicillin coming off quicker than I could count them. It was then I knew that the battle had been won and that victory was ours. It had been a long road from Fleming's petri dish to the finished vials, ready for the physicians' hands."

While the war indirectly contributed to the production of penicillin being transferred to the United States (many in the United Kingdom still accuse America of stealing penicillin, which they regard as uniquely British, even though Florey was Australian and Chain was a German Jew who had fled to England to escape from the rising Hitler regime), it was also the theater in which the greatest early successes with the drug were seen, and which unquestionably propelled it to megastar status. During World War I, 15 percent of those wounded in battle had died of infection. The sulfa drugs, introduced before the Second World War, had initially had a remarkable impact in reducing battle casualties, but nothing compared with what was achieved with penicillin. Open fractures, particularly vulnerable to life-threatening osteomyelitis, showed a recovery of close to 100 percent. There were thousands of case reports of burned soldiers making complete recoveries. None of this would have been possible without penicillin. The age of antibiotics had begun.

CHAPTER 9

More Cures and the Widening Problem

Despite never having purified penicillin nor having directly saved even one life with it, Fleming was penicillin's champion, never losing his optimism for its therapeutic potential during a period when many of his medical colleagues were skeptical. Had Fleming abandoned his research, undoubtedly someone else would have eventually discovered it, but the delay would have cost millions of lives. For this alone, Fleming is deserving of all the fame history has heaped upon him, even though he wasn't even the first to discover what we now call an antibiotic. Medical practices employing products remarkably similar to what modern science uses today had, in fact, been with us for millennia.

More than four thousand years ago the Chinese routinely treated skin wounds and infections with a paste made from moldy soybeans. Almost identical remedies are described in the Hebrew Talmud. As recounted by Dr. Mark Lappé in his 1982 book, *Germs That Won't Die*, a hieroglyphic on an Egyptian column from the year 2160 B.C. depicts a physician giving a cup of beer to a high priest. Legend has it that the beer was used to mask the extremely bitter taste of the herbal preparations the Egyptian physicians used as medicines.

The ancient practices all had as a common denominator the use of fermented grains, with molds, yeast and fungi as the fermenting agents. Until the 1960s, when scientists at pharmaceutical companies began developing synthetic versions of antibiotics, the naturally produced ones were derived from similar sources: molds, sewage or soil. As the bacteria or fungi producing these early antibiotics have been around for millions of years, it is likely that the pastes, packs or liquids used by these early healers contained antibiotics in some form.

More solid substantiation of this was uncovered recently by a team of archaeologists working on a dig in Sudan. They excavated the remains of a Nubian civilization believed to have been in existence around 350 A.D., and when they decalcified and chemically analyzed some of the human bones, they found trace evidence of the antibiotic tetracycline. Since the tetracycline was recovered from the bones, it indicated that the antibiotic had been ingested, metabolized and then deposited in the skeleton. The source of the tetracycline appeared to be the soil bacteria *Streptomyces,* the same source from which Benjamin Duggar isolated tetracycline at Lederle laboratories in Pearl River, New York, almost sixteen hundred years later. Presumably, the bacteria contaminated the bins where grains were stored and from which the bread this civilization ate as a daily staple was subsequently made. What we don't know is whether the tetracycline-producing bacteria were ingested by these ancient people intentionally or accidentally. Because the Nubian civilization survived until the fourteenth century, far longer than any other people who lived in that area of the world at that time, some anthropologists have concluded that the Nubians probably had a much lower incidence of infectious disease than neighboring societies did. It is entirely plausible that Nubian physicians correctly attributed certain therapeutic properties to the contaminated grains and made certain that most of the bread consumed was made from them.

In *Miracle Cure,* Milton Wainwright describes a similar practice that began in England in the seventeenth century. John Parkinson, the apothecary of London and the king's herbalist, recommended the use of moldy bread to treat infected wounds. Wainwright also makes mention of a letter written to the *Sunday Express* on March 19, 1989, by a minister who said that penicillin had been used in several parts of Yorkshire for more than one hundred years. It was the custom there on Good Friday to bake hot cross buns, he wrote, but housewives always intentionally prepared more than the family would be able to eat. The leftover buns were put away in a special tin container and deliberately allowed to turn moldy. Later, the buns were removed from what were in effect mini–antibiotic factories, the mold was scraped into a jar, incorporated into an ointment and then used for the remainder of the year as a highly effective topical treatment for superficial cuts and abrasions.

Molds as anti-infective agents were also used by the American Indians. In what must have seemed like magic to him, in 1911 an American physician in North Carolina named John Bricknell observed an Indian witch doctor cure an infected leg ulcer by applying a powder that he had made by grinding up moldy kernels of Indian corn.

Although we should look back on the resourcefulness of these ancient medical practitioners with amazed admiration, their therapies were obviously crude and employed entirely on an empirical basis. None of these folk healers had the slightest idea what was actually causing the infections they were treating or why the treatments worked. And there is no evidence that Fleming or his contemporaries were in any way influenced by, or even knew of, any of these primitive customs. Fleming certainly never referred to them in his writings or lectures, nor would he have even if he had been aware of the rich medical culture that had preceded his work. Fleming was a scientist, and for a Western scientist in those times (or for that matter in these times) to have given even the slightest credence to the practices of witch doctors and medicine men would have made him an immediate laughingstock and certainly been cause for dismissal from the Royal Society.

The real scientific thread to which Fleming, other microbial scientists and all antibiotics are attached began near the end of the nineteenth century. By 1870, medical science had in many ways become advanced. Anatomy taught in medical schools wasn't much different from what aspiring doctors learn today. Physiology and pharmacology were becoming well-respected scientific disciplines. But the treatment of infectious diseases lagged behind miserably and was hardly more sophisticated than in the time of the ancient Egyptians. People died in droves from pneumonia, cholera, tuberculosis, scarlet fever and typhoid, and physicians were at almost a complete loss in treating or preventing infectious diseases. The only progress that had been made could be counted on a few fingers: Semmelweis's demonstration that regular hand-washing reduced the spread of childbirth fever, Joseph Lister's discovery that using a carbolic acid spray in surgery could help prevent postoperative infections, and Edward Jenner's use of the cowpox virus to immunize against smallpox. If any of these preventive measures failed, however, and they often did, physicians had nothing left in their black bags.

The main reason for this dismal rate of success was that the cause of the infections was still a mystery. Scientists did know that bacteria existed. This had been demonstrated more than two hundred years earlier in the Netherlands by Anton van Leeuwenhoek, who wasn't even a scientist but a merchant. He was also, however, an inventor, and while tinkering at home he devised the world's first microscope, a primitive but elegant hand-held set of lenses. In 1674, he peered with his new instrument into a drop of water and discovered a whole new world. He called the tiny creatures he observed "wee animalcules," and sent detailed descriptions and drawings to the Royal Society in London, which opened eyes but not minds. What he was observing, of course, were bacteria, and while the members of the Royal Society welcomed Leeuwenhoek's contribution to the body of knowledge, there was virtually no significance attached to his observations. These little beings were a mere scientific curiosity and remained just that for a long time. It would be more than two centuries before any connection between these microorganisms and disease would be made.

The one most responsible for making this connection was Louis Pasteur, a scientist whose name is far more recognizable than even Fleming's, and rightly so, for it was Pasteur's work that finally took both the diagnosis and treatment of infectious diseases out of the Middle Ages and began to blaze the trail that would eventually lead Fleming to penicillin.

Until Pasteur's work, it was generally believed that microorganisms arose by a process called spontaneous generation; that is, they magically emerged de novo from inanimate matter. Pasteur, however, never believed this. He was convinced that in regard to how they were produced, microorganisms were no different from human beings. Bacteria could arise only from other bacteria. At his laboratory in Paris, he devised a magnificent set of experiments to show that the microorganisms found on spoiling meat or rotting flesh came from the air, settled into the tissues and multiplied, eventually causing the tissues to decay. This refutation of spontaneous generation was corroborated in England by the Victorian mathematician and physicist John Tyndall. (A small cadre of historians also believe that during these experiments Tyndall may actually have stumbled on penicillin, and they believe its discovery should be attributed to him instead of Fleming. But since he did not follow up his observations, Fleming's reputation seems safe.)

Pasteur's observations eventually led him in the 1870s to far greater understanding of the growth and metabolism of microorganisms than had ever been achieved and to the accomplishments for which he is most remembered. He was able to explain how bread rises, how milk and other food spoils and, of great importance to the French economy, how wine is made. But it was with his germ theory of disease, in which he hypothesized that bacteria invading live tissue and multiplying were the cause of most infections, that Pasteur undoubtedly made his greatest contribution to humankind.

Then, in 1881, Robert Koch, a German physician, made two additional important discoveries. Working in his kitchen with a potato extract, he developed an agar-gelatin mixture. He was then able to get bacteria to adhere to the sticky surface of this mixture and grow into well-defined colonies for further study. With only minor variations over the past one hundred years, this same mixture is still used in virtually every hospital microbiology laboratory in the world to grow and isolate bacteria from specimens of urine, blood, sputum and other tissues and fluids.

The ability to grow bacteria allowed Koch to perform experiments that otherwise wouldn't have been possible. In proving that the bacterium *Mycobacterium tuberculosis* was the cause of tuberculosis, he developed the series of conditions that every medical student learns must be satisfied to establish an organism as the causative agent of a disease. Called Koch's postulates, they are:

- The microorganism must be present in every case of the disease
- It must be capable of cultivation in pure culture
- When inoculated from this culture, it must produce the disease in susceptible animals
- It must be able to be recovered from these diseased animals and grown again in pure culture

Pasteur's germ theory of disease and Koch's work truly revolutionized medicine. Researchers today are identifying new genes at an accelerated rate, but Pasteur and others began to recognize and name new bacteria at a remarkably comparable pace. As a consequence of this early systematic identification, by the mid-1880s many diseases that until then had eluded analysis finally began to shed their cloaks of mystery.

For the first time, it became possible to link a specific condition and set of symptoms with one of the new kinds of bacteria. Scientists learned that by taking specimens from patients, such as throat swabs or urine specimens or sputum, the bacteria that grew out on Koch's agar would form colonies with easily defined and reproducible morphology. And using the microscope, which by then had become quite sophisticated, it was discovered that bacteria observed under magnification had even more defining characteristics.

The ability to do this was enhanced considerably as a result of a chance observation made in 1881 by a Danish scientist, Hans Christian Gram. Gram was a pathologist and was working with a variety of dyes in an attempt to stain and therefore highlight damage in tissue specimens. He noticed that some bacteria in these tissues "held" a purple dye he had been using, while it was easily washed off of others, which could then be stained with a pink dye. Using this simple technique, it became possible to classify all bacteria as either gram-positive (those that held the purple stain) or gram-negative (those that didn't hold the purple stain but subsequently held the pink stain). Although it was not known at the time, because the ability or inability to hold the stain is dependent on the characteristics of the bacterial cell wall, the Gram stain would eventually be used as a differentiating point in determining which antibiotics would be effective against which kinds of bacteria.

But even without this understanding, the Gram stain still proved immensely valuable. Once the bacteria were stained, it became easier to study other characteristics of their structure, the most important of which was whether they were rod-shaped (called bacilli) or sphere-shaped (cocci). This led to the development of an entire new terminology and compendium of disease-causing bacteria. Gram-positive cocci that tended to grow primarily in chains were called streptococci (Greek *streptos* = twisted), and it was observed time after time that these streptococci were isolated from patients with sore throats or scarlet fever. Gram-positive cocci that grew in pairs were called diplococci (*di* = two), and it was discovered that these were often isolated from patients with pneumonia. (The association later became so constant that the name was eventually changed to pneumococcus, to reflect the disease the bacteria caused rather than their microscopic morphology.) Gram-positive cocci that grew mainly in clusters were called staphylococci (Greek *staphyl* = grapes), and it was found that these bacteria were regularly isolated from severe blood poisoning, boils, abscesses and certain types of pneumonia.

Being aware of which bacteria did what and what they looked like made it easier for pathologists to decipher just how they cause disease and how our bodies defend us against them. In most cases, nature has made it difficult for us to contract a bacterial infection. Only a small fraction of bacteria that exist are pathogenic to humans; the remainder are harmless or sometimes even helpful to us. Even for those types that can cause disease, it normally takes a concentrated invasion of the offending microorganism; usually at least a thousand and in some cases as many as a million bacteria are required before any damage is done. The most glaring exception to this rule is tuberculosis, where, if conditions are just right, only one tubercule bacillus can lead to disease.

For our part, we have developed an elaborate and multitiered network of protection against foreign invaders. It begins with the skin, which acts as the largest barrier to bacterial entry, but one that is purely a physical impediment. If the integrity of the skin is broken, a ready portal is provided for microorganisms to scurry through and establish themselves. Another defense is the numerous mucous membranes of our body—those that line our mouth, our nose, our intestines and our genital tracts. The deterrent here isn't just a physical obstacle but rather the slippery secretions produced by the cells lining these areas which make it difficult for bacteria to adhere and multiply. In addition, our nose, which is so exposed to the outside environment and which is the gatekeeper to our lungs, has another protective device called cilia, tiny hairs that beat constantly in a wavelike motion to propel any bacteria that might enter the nasal passages away from the lower respiratory tract.

If bacteria do get by these obstacles, they meet up with the most sophisticated and dedicated component of our defense against infectious disease: the white blood cells and the rest of the immune system. Some white blood cells act as sentries and are able to engulf and digest bacteria. Others produce antibodies, specific proteins that, like a torpedo with a heat-seeking head, lock in on the bacteria and immobilize them, allowing other white blood cells to come along and transport the bacteria to lymph nodes or to the spleen, where they are destroyed.

With all these defenses, the odds are stacked very much against bacteria ever gaining enough of a foothold in our bodies to cause disease. Even in those rare instances when we are exposed to pathogenic bacteria, our immune police force is so efficient that we aren't even aware there has been a bacterial incursion. When the bacteria do succeed in causing a disease, it is because of either a breakdown in our defenses, such as a cut in the skin, or, more important, a malfunction or suppression of our immune system. Sometimes, however, it is because of some intrinsic properties of the bacteria themselves.

Early on, Pasteur and then his scientific heirs observed that bacteria whose cell walls are rough are not as virulent as those whose cells walls are smooth. The sentry white blood cells responsible for engulfing the bacteria have less of a handle to grab on to when they encounter smooth invaders, so the bacteria are more likely to slip by at least one arm of the defense system. Most pathogenic bacteria have a variety of other tricks up their sleeve. Just as cancer cells have developed structural means of avoiding detection by the immune cells, so have bacteria (actually, the bacteria probably developed them first). By changing just a few sequences in their biochemical processes, they are able to don a molecular disguise that makes them look for all the world like one of the cells of the organism they invaded. In other cases, the bacteria make it difficult for the white blood cells to ingest them, even if they can be detected and grabbed hold of. Finally, there are some bacteria, such as the tuberculosis bacteria and *Mycoplasma,* that are not destroyed when they are being ingested by the white blood cells; they actually thrive inside them. This is similar to the way HIV survives and multiplies.

If the bacteria are able to evade our defenses, they then settle in the location most conducive to their survival. To establish themselves, the most pathogenic bacteria then use another arrow in their quiver and secrete substances that allow them to attach to the cells of the organ they have invaded. Given a sufficient supply of nutrients, most bacteria are capable of reproducing themselves every twenty minutes, so within a short period of time—as short as only one day—there can be a whole colony. As they grow, they invade further into the tissues, often producing enzymes that destroy the integrity of the organ even more. If the microorganisms are particularly aggressive and if the immune system they have successfully evaded in getting to this point doesn't recover quickly enough to mount a second-line attack and limit the damage, the end result is often death—that is, until we discovered antibiotics.

A rational search for antibacterial agents, substances that would enhance our own defenses, was the most important outgrowth of the germ theory of disease. Physicians began this hunt almost immediately. And, not surprisingly, the first to discover something significant was Pasteur, in a set of circumstances that preceded Fleming's by some fifty years, but which were remarkably similar in their sequence. The only difference was that, on this occasion, Pasteur uncharacteristically fumbled. He had grown some anthrax bacteria—one of the first type of bacteria ever isolated and known to be responsible for a serious disease, primarily in animals—and noticed that his bacterial culture was contaminated. He was astute and interested enough, however, not to throw the plate away, instead incubating it overnight. The next day, he discovered that the bacteria had been completely destroyed by the contaminating culture.

Pasteur did immediately recognize that this sort of microbial antagonism—one bacterium or fungus with the ability to kill another—had tremendous import for the therapy of disease. So what he did next was inject the anthrax bacteria into guinea pigs and follow that with injections of a wide variety of soil bacteria. He found that some of the soil bacteria were actually able to protect the guinea pigs from anthrax. But where he made his mistake was in not isolating the contaminating organism responsible for killing the anthrax bacteria. Had he done so, he might have discovered penicillin a half century before Fleming.

Pasteur's observations were not lost, however. Other scientists began to pick up on the notion of microbial antagonism. One of them, the German scientist Rudolph Emmerich, along with his colleague Oscar Loew, showed in 1899 that the residues of cultures of a bacterium called *Pseudomonas pyocyanea* were able to protect guinea pigs from diphtheria, and then from anthrax and typhoid. Unlike Pasteur, Emmerich determined which bacteria were responsible for creating the antagonism, and he also succeeded in isolating the substance responsible for the effect. He named it pyocyanase. Although few of us have ever heard of it, pyocyanase was actually the first antibiotic to be identified. It was also the first to be commercially produced. Excitement over Emmerich's discovery so infected the medical community that within just two years pyocyanase was being manufactured in several countries on the European continent. Unfortunately, pyocyanase proved to be a painful reminder of the fact that what works in the lab doesn't always work on people. Within just a couple of years after production was in full swing, there was a swarm of reports of both toxicity with pyocyanase and its failure to cure patients. Even though it continued to be used, mostly topically, for another ten years or so, pyocyanase was essentially dead.

Another German scientist, a contemporary of Pasteur's, took a slightly different approach, working with synthetic chemicals rather than living microorganisms. This path laid the foundation for a huge breakthrough. The scientist was Paul Ehrlich, a true scientific giant, the acknowledged father of both immunology and chemotherapy. During his medical residency at Charite Hospital in Berlin in 1881, Ehrlich had published a paper on the use of the dye methylene blue as a bacterial stain. It was a different stain from the one devised by

Gram and never gained wide application in bacterial identification. But it wasn't in identification that Ehrlich believed methylene blue would have its greatest use. The dye stained and killed the bacteria because of its affinity for them, which he thought could be of value in the therapy of disease. The concept, that specific chemicals could kill microorganisms without harming the host—a magic bullet— was revolutionary. Ehrlich's idea in 1881 was the birth of the specific chemotherapy of disease. Although it focuses on the elimination of tumor cells rather than bacteria, the chemotherapy of cancer is the result of this simple experiment Ehrlich performed with methylene blue dye.

Chemotherapy, however, is also widely used in the treatment of infections, and Ehrlich persisted with this notion, although he was interrupted for several years, first by contracting tuberculosis and then by his work on immunology, which eventually earned him the Nobel Prize. In the late 1890s, Ehrlich returned to methylene blue and attempted to use it for the treatment of malaria. He noticed that the tuberculosis bacteria were intensely stained by the dye, and he convinced his friend and former teacher Robert Koch (who had earlier used methylene blue to help him identify the tuberculosis bacterium) to try methylene blue in cases of malaria that proved recalcitrant to quinine, the only available therapy. There were actually some early successes, but just as Emmerich had found with his bacterial substance, Ehrlich's chemical proved too toxic and too ineffective to be used widely. Ehrlich, however, was not dissuaded from his fascination with methylene blue. He boldly predicted that, if other related chemicals could be tried, eventually a highly effective and relatively nontoxic one would be found. Thirty years later, his prediction came true with the introduction of quinacrine (Atabrine), still today one of the most effective antimalarial compounds.

Ehrlich did achieve success working with another group of chemicals, the arsenicals (derived from arsenic). At first he used them to treat parasitic conditions and later decided to test the arsenicals in his lab in an experimental model of syphilis in rabbits. After seemingly endless trials, one compound, number 606 in the series, proved extraordinarily effective. Human trials followed, and in 1910, compound 606, or Salvarsan, as it was known, became the first drug ever used to treat syphilis, albeit not without some devastating toxic side effects (which drew biting criticism from many sources, including the *Journal of the American Medical Association* in a 1914 article). But it was difficult to criticize the almost miraculous cures achieved with Salvarsan. Patients practically stormed the factory in the town of Hoechst, where the drug was being manufactured, demanding to be treated. Within just five years after widespread use of Salvarsan began, the incidence of syphilis in England and France had decreased by 50 percent. Ehrlich died a few years later of a recurrence of his tuberculosis.

The stunning success with Salvarsan, despite the problems, convinced scientists that other magic bullets could be developed. And because Salvarsan had proven far more effective than pyocyanase, the only frame of reference, for the moment the synthetic chemical approach rather than a search for natural compounds produced by microorganisms was more in vogue. Even with concentrated effort in this direction, however, it was to be two more decades before another suitable chemical compound could be found.

Success again came in Germany, at IG Farbenindustrie, the huge chemical conglomerate which became known not only for innovations in the chemotherapy of infections but for the development of synthetic oil, a breakthrough which at least for a time aided the Nazi war effort. The research on infections at Farben took place at its Bayer subsidiary (the recently acquired company that had first synthesized aspirin) and was a direct descendant of Ehrlich's work. The approach was to synthesize chemical compounds and then test them for antibacterial activity. An enormous number of these compounds were developed, and a huge screening operation was set up to test them.

This sort of approach was criticized by many academicians, especially Sir Almoth Wright, Alexander Fleming's boss at St. Mary's Hospital. Wright, who only a few years earlier had opposed Fleming's research on penicillin, believed that a better and safer way to battle bacterial invaders was from the other side of the equation—by stimulating the patient's white blood cells and increasing resistance. Wright had been invited to visit IG Farben and, after touring the facility, made caustic comments to his colleagues about the German setup. One of them described his reaction as follows: "He regaled us at tea with the story that he had been shown enormous laboratories in which they did nothing but take compound after compound and test its ability to deal with infections in animals caused by a variety of organisms. Blind groping in the dark in this way was so utterly foreign to someone of Wright's temperament that he looked upon it as a form of sacrilege."

Had Wright delayed his trip to Germany, he might have had a different opinion of the Bayer method, because it was soon to reap results. In the early 1930s, Gerhard Domagk, the director of research, set up an experimental model of streptococcal infections in mice and began to test a variety of compounds, using the mass screening system in place. The compounds he would use were those that had shown some antibacterial activity in the test tube. For some reason, however, in one set of experiments Domagk decided to include a group of compounds called azo dyes, even though they had shown absolutely no antibacterial activity when previously tested. It is now believed that he was following Ehrlich's reasoning that if dyes stained tissues they might be of some use in preventing bacterial penetration. And he turned out to be right. One of the azo dyes, the red dye Prontosil, proved enormously effective in curing streptococcal infections in mice. French collaborators discovered shortly thereafter that the activity of Prontosil resided in the portion of the molecule called sulfonamide. And because sulfonamide was released only when the dye was injected into an animal, it explained why Prontosil was inactive in the test tube. Domagk had done the important work, but it was Paul Ehrlich's legacy that had led him to the sulfa drugs.

There was no comparison between the importance of the sulfa drugs and the magic bullets that had preceded them. Here was finally a compound that physicians could use effectively without risking their patients' lives, or even any serious side effects. Pyocyanase and Salvarsan were virtually forgotten. With the sulfa drugs, still used to treat certain infections today, we had entered the antimicrobial era, never to turn back. Even penicillin was a beneficiary. Following the initial successes with sulfa drugs in the mid-1930s, efforts to purify penicillin were stepped up, with triumph to come only a few years later. And when the effectiveness of penicillin overshadowed even the sulfa drugs, research shifted from the synthetic chemicals to natural antimicrobial compounds.

There was also a geographical shift, across the Atlantic to the United States, where streptomycin, the world's second major effective antibiotic, was discovered. The credit for that discovery is generally given to Selman Waksman, and to Waksman alone, an accomplishment for which he too was to receive the Nobel Prize. It was Waksman who coined the term "antibiotic" in 1941, in a letter to the editor of the journal *Biologic Abstracts*, as the appropriate name for a compound made by one microorganism that inhibits the growth of another. This definition still holds today and is the reason why sulfa drugs, which are synthesized chemically rather than naturally derived, are technically not antibiotics, but instead are called antimicrobials.

The story of streptomycin has been less publicized than that of penicillin, yet the details surrounding its discovery are no less fascinating. Just like Fleming, Waksman was pretty far along in his career when he took an interest in microbial antagonism, yet he approached it from an entirely different perspective.

Waksman was born in Russia in 1888 and emigrated to the United States in 1910. Although he had been a brilliant young student, showing great scientific aptitude, there was a wave of anti-Semitism in Russia, and consequently Waksman was denied a formal university education. When he first arrived in the United States, he supported himself by working on his cousin's farm, and developed a keen interest in agriculture and the soil. He enrolled at Rutgers University, where he obtained an undergraduate and a graduate degree. Later he earned a doctorate at the University of California. In 1918 he returned to Rutgers as a lecturer and became interested in microbial antagonism, not for its therapeutic potential but rather to learn more about how bacteria and fungi interact in the soil, a passion he pursued for more than twenty years.

In the early 1940s, Waksman heard about the success with penicillin, and then became convinced that the soil could yield many other antibiotics. He set up a "shotgun approach," sampling as many soils as possible and screening them for antimicrobial activity, first in the test tube and then in animal experiments. Within only a short time, Waksman's hunch was borne out when he and his colleagues isolated two antibiotics, streptothricin and actinomycin. Both proved too toxic for general human use (actinomycin, however, found application in the chemotherapy of cancer and is still used today), but the principle had been demonstrated. They were convinced it would be only a matter of time before they found the right compound.

And just a couple of years later, Waksman and his team indeed hit pay dirt when they isolated streptomycin from two different strains of the soil bacteria *Actinomyces,* the same bacteria that earlier had yielded the too-toxic antibiotics. One of Waksman's graduate students, Albert Schatz, actually did the lion's share of the work on the new compound, not only isolating it from samples of the bacteria, but also rigorously performing efficacy and toxicity tests. He wrote up the results in his doctoral thesis in 1945.

A year earlier, however, the research team had published a paper in *The Proceedings of the Society for Experimental Biology and Medicine* titled "Streptomycin: A Substance Exhibiting Antibiotic Activity Against Gram-Positive and Gram-Negative Bacteria." Although Waksman allowed Schatz's name to appear first on the paper, he gave his brilliant student little credit, later calling him nothing more than a "pair of hands." It was the beginning of an acrimonious relationship between mentor and pupil, which resulted in Schatz leaving Rutgers a few years later, accusing Waksman of stealing streptomycin royalties from him (which he apparently did, although he put most of the money back into the Rutgers microbiology department) and eventually filing a lawsuit against Waksman. The scientific community sided almost unanimously with the now famous professor, and Rutgers, embarrassed by the legal action, essentially purged the name of Albert Schatz from its publicity department. And so did Waksman. In a later autobiography, *My Life with the Microbes,* he made not one mention of Schatz.

Aside from the personal controversy it generated, the 1944 paper created tremendous excitement in the scientific community. Except for those who could see what was coming, cases of penicillin resistance were not yet numerous enough to dampen enthusiasm for the drug even slightly. But penicillin did have one inherent shortcoming of which all physicians and scientists were aware: with only a few exceptions, it was effective only against gram-positive bacteria.

Ever since Robert Koch had identified the causative organism more than fifty years earlier, the world had been waiting and hoping for a cure for TB. By 1937, tuberculosis was the number one cause of death in the United States and, when penicillin was first introduced, it was hailed by tuberculosis patients as a savior. But penicillin couldn't touch the organisms that caused the disease.

When it was stated in Schatz and Waksman's paper that streptomycin was able to kill gram-negative bacteria, as well as *Mycobacterium tuberculosis*, a cure was once again eagerly anticipated. But it was already known that the tuberculosis bacillus was a tricky organism to kill. Before climbing that mountain, Waksman suggested demonstrating streptomycin's mettle against more conventional gram-negative bacteria, all of which had been immune to penicillin therapy. These included meningococcal meningitis, *Salmonella* infections, intestinal infections caused by *Shigella*, and infections with bacteria called *Klebsiella*, referred to by most physicians as "walking pneumonia." Early clinical trials with streptomycin against these diseases were so successful that the pharmaceutical company Merck set up a huge facility in Rahway, New Jersey, just down the road from New Brunswick and Waksman's laboratory at Rutgers, dedicated to the production of the new antibiotic. Whether or not streptomycin would prove valuable in treating tuberculosis, it was already felt that it would be an important treatment for a whole range of infectious diseases caused by gram-negative bacteria.

In fact, streptomycin was also successful in treating tuberculosis. Its first administration was on November 15, 1945, to a twenty-one-year-old patient at the Mineral Springs Sanatorium in Canon Falls, Minnesota. Despite having far-advanced pulmonary tuberculosis, she experienced a miraculous recovery. When reevaluated in 1954, nine years after her treatment, she was still healthy, had married and had three children. As her physician wrote in a 1955 article in the *American Review of Tuberculosis,* "The streptomycin which this patient received in the first clinical trial of the drug was definitely beneficial and may even have been lifesaving. It is a happy ending which has been duplicated tens of thousands of times in the streptomycin story."

But such enthusiasm ignored two major problems that developed with streptomycin treatment of tuberculosis. In animal trials, and the early human clinical trials, streptomycin had been remarkably nontoxic. In order to cure tuberculosis, however, high doses of the antibiotic were required, and at these high doses, toxic side effects surfaced. Most of them involved the inner and middle ear, beginning with tinnitus, or ringing in the ears, followed by vertigo, loss of balance and in some cases total deafness. All of these complications were due to the action of a metabolic by-product of streptomycin on the auditory nerve and proved irreversible. While doctors were not strangers to the toxic effects of a drug, the two antibacterial compounds that had preceded streptomycin, sulfa drugs and penicillin, were so devoid of toxic effects that they were taken by surprise. The side effects of streptomycin were clearly dose-related and by lowering the amount given to patients, many diseases could still be cured without side effects. Unfortunately, when the dose was lowered, tuberculosis wasn't remedied.

The main reason such a high dose of streptomycin was needed was because of the other problem. The tuberculosis bacteria developed resistance to the antibiotic at an astonishing rate, greater than anything that had been experienced with penicillin. In 1946 came a report from Northwestern University that the amount of streptomycin required to kill the tuberculosis bacteria increased as much as a thousand times during therapy. This resistance was due to a fatal combination of bacteria and an antibiotic, each with unique properties. Few bacteria have been studied that display an ability to become resistant to any antibiotic as rapidly as *Mycobacterium tuberculosis*. And even fifty years and hundreds of antibiotics later, streptomycin still stands as the antibiotic to which any bacteria are most likely to become resistant.

The silver lining was that resistance to streptomycin led to the first use of combination antimicrobial therapy, routinely employed today not only for tuberculosis but for other diseases. The theory, which proved to be true, was that adding other drugs to streptomycin would decrease the ability of the tubercle bacillus to become resistant to any of them. The two that were added were PAS and isoniazid, the latter of which was first produced by Dr. Domagk, the inventor of sulfa drugs. Although streptomycin is rarely used in most industrialized countries anymore to treat tuberculosis (having been replaced by rifampin, which is derived from the same soil bacteria as streptomycin), this combination was effective for many years and is estimated to have reduced the death rates in the United States by two-thirds. Despite the problems of toxicity and resistance, streptomycin had to be considered a major success.

At this point in the discovery and development of antibiotics, the American pharmaceutical companies began to be proactive rather than reactive. The seminal work on penicillin and streptomycin had been done at academic institutions and later mass-produced and marketed with the help of Merck, Pfizer and other drug companies. But now, realizing the enormous economic potential, these companies turned their research departments largely into screening programs for antibiotics, much as had been done in Germany at IG Farbenindustrie. Whether or not it was a demonstration that the profit incentive was a stronger motivator to antibiotic discovery than altruism, the next fifteen years were the most fruitful period in antibiotic history, and are still referred to as the "golden age of antibiotics." The first of the drugs to originate from this pipeline was chloramphenicol at Parke Davis in 1947, followed by chlortetracycline at Lederle in 1948 and then erythromycin (1952), vancomycin (1956), methicillin (1961) and gentamicin (1963). There have been many others since then, of course, but each of these earlier drugs represents an important biochemical achievement from which many of the later antibiotics were derived.

Our story of antibiotic discovery and development would not be complete, however, without a brief description of how the most commonly used group of antibiotics today, the cephalosporins, came into being. Cephalosporin is unique not only in that it was one of the few antibiotics that wasn't discovered in the United States, England or Germany but also because of the source of the fungus that was originally found to produce it.

Giuseppe Brotzu, a professor of bacteriology at Cagliari University on the island of Sardinia, had an idea that was an outgrowth of Waksman's search for antibiotics in soil bacteria. Since the bacteria that cause typhoid fever are so commonly found in sewage, he reasoned that there might have developed a source of a compound antagonistic to them that might also be found in sewage. He spent several months at what had to be the least attractive spot on beautiful Sardinia, at a local sewage outlet, collecting material just as it was discharged into the sea and isolating microorganisms. His painstaking work resulted in the isolation of the fungus that produces cephalosporin. It would take almost twenty years before the material could be purified enough (with help from Florey and Chain, who had become purification masters) for therapeutic application. But just as Fleming deserves the credit for penicillin, so does Brotzu deserve it for cephalosporin. To date there have been three generations and dozens of these compounds introduced. In their present iteration, they are capable of treating virtually every type of bacterium. And although the flow is slowing, there are still more cephalosporins in the pipeline.

But just as with all the other antibiotics, resistance to the cephalosporins did develop and has been increasing. And once again, the question must be asked: Will these latest miracle drugs become tomorrow's plague makers? Unfortunately, this is likely to be what happens.

CHAPTER 10

The Miseducation of Physicians

It is three A.M. on a typical hectic Saturday night in the emergency department of a large university teaching hospital. Every bed is filled with critically ill patients, from gunshot wounds to car wrecks to drug overdoses. Doctors, nurses, radiology technicians and lab personnel are practically bumping into one another, rushing from one room to another. Suddenly, another ambulance pulls up outside the ER door and the paramedics hurriedly wheel in a stretcher carrying an elderly woman in obvious pain. Despite being in the midst of suturing another patient, the closest doctor reflexively strips off his latex gloves and runs to her side. The woman is sweating and ashen with a weak, rapid pulse; her breathing is labored. The tracing on the electrocardiogram taken by the paramedics indicates she has had an acute anterior myocardial infarction (heart attack).

After connecting her to the appropriate monitoring equipment and quickly assessing her condition, the doctors unanimously decide that the patient's symptoms are severe enough to warrant emergency cardiac catheterization to look for the site of blockage in her coronary arteries. During the procedure, she experiences an abnormal heart rhythm, necessitating the insertion of a balloon pump into her aorta. These heroics stabilize the patient's condition enough so that she can be returned to the cardiac intensive care unit. Seemingly she is out of the woods, but her biggest troubles are about to begin.

The admitting nurse in the ICU notices her patient is now running a high fever and that her blood pressure is low. A chest x-ray taken in the operating room indicates fluid buildup in her lungs. The nurse summons the medical resident on duty, and the young doctor studies the chart and examines her new patient. In her mind, she quickly sifts through a differential diagnosis. Probably congestive heart failure secondary to the heart attack, she assumes. But what if the patient has a pneumonia on top of everything else? She decides to play it safe and start treating with some antibiotics.

After taking samples of sputum and blood, which are promptly sent to the laboratory for bacterial culture, the doctor thinks again. She vaguely remembers having heard just last week something about the latest cephalosporin antibiotic, and that it was being touted as a new and highly effective treatment for pneumonia. Silently congratulating herself on her cutting-edge information, she instructs the nurse to order some of this new antibiotic from the hospital pharmacy and then give it to the patient intravenously every four hours. About to walk away, the doctor has an afterthought and adds an antibiotic called clindamycin to her orders, to protect against the possibility that any pneumonia might be caused by anaerobic bacteria (those that grow only in the absence of oxygen). Feeling secure after having ordered this drug regimen, the resident turns her attention to her other patients.

During rounds the next day, the patient appears better. Her blood pressure has stabilized, her pulse has slowed and her breathing is more regular. The chief resident compliments his protégée on her handling of the case. But the patient's fever persists and so does some fluid in her lungs. When the resident calls the lab for the results of the cultures, she is told there has been no bacterial growth. The radiologist reports that the opacities seen on chest x-ray are almost certainly not pneumonia.

Unsure how to proceed, the medical resident consults with the infectious disease resident. With an air of authority, he disregards the negative laboratory and x-ray reports and immediately recommends adding another powerful antibiotic, vancomycin. One day later during a residents' conference, without even seeing the patient, the chief of the medical service tells the young doctor to add yet two more expensive and broad-spectrum antibiotics, ticarcillin–clavulanic acid and tobramycin, "to give better coverage for gram-negative bacteria." Four days later, the patient develops septicemia (blood poisoning). More heroic measures are tried, including additional antibiotics. Despite this, the patient dies within two days. Postmortem blood cultures indicate the cause of death was a massive overgrowth of yeast in her blood.

In many of the best hospitals in the United States, a case like this occurs repeatedly, practically every day. On the surface, it may have the earmarks of sophisticated, well-thought-out medical care. And the care was first-rate in the emergency room and in surgery. But after that it was anything but well thought out. The alphabet soup of antibiotics given to this patient is a perfect example of how irrationally and inappropriately these drugs have come to be used, and how little logic permeates the decisions of many of even the most educated doctors.

The purpose of antibiotics is simple: they are supposed to be used to treat documented bacterial infections, ones in which the causative organism has been properly identified. But we have come so far from that axiom, it's almost as if it never existed. Instead, doctors treat more and more diseases empirically, either without waiting for or ignoring laboratory results of cultures of blood, sputum or other body fluids.

Sometimes, if a patient is critically ill, an empiric approach is justified, but then only for a short time, until the patient responds positively or the results of the microbial cultures are available. In one sense, the medical resident in this case was using sound judgment in beginning her patient on the two antibiotics. Pneumonia *was* a real possibility and the benefits of beginning therapy before there was objective evidence of infection outweighed the risks. But the doctor's choice of the antibiotics was not based on informed objectivity. One of them was selected on the assumption that if a drug was new it must be the right one. The other was chosen to give "shotgun" coverage to the patient, even though the chances of any pneumonia being caused by anaerobic bacteria were remote.

And medical wisdom went out the window completely when the reports of the negative cultures and the essentially negative radiology report were returned. At that point, not only should the infectious disease resident have insisted that no more antibiotics be added, but also that the first two be discontinued and the patient be treated for mild congestive heart failure. In this case, the continued use of antibiotics had two devastating effects. Besides contributing to the global pool of resistant bacteria, there were fatal consequences for the individual patient. Elderly and ill with a suppressed immune system, she almost certainly died of an overwhelming yeast infection because the several broad-spectrum antibiotics her doctors administered had killed off all competition and allowed the opportunistic *Candida* to grow.

The use of antibiotics this inappropriately goes well beyond empiric therapy. It has been called "spiraling empiricism" by Dr. James E. Peacock of Bowman-Gray School of Medicine (Wake Forest University) and Dr. Harry Gallis, chief of infectious diseases at Duke University School of Medicine. And spiraling empiricism doesn't just involve critically ill patients. In terms of selecting for resistant strains of bacteria, the same irrational and dangerous principles are also at work when your doctor prescribes an antibiotic for a cold or minor sore throat.

Why are such poor decisions made? Why are antibiotics given so carelessly? One reason, mentioned earlier, is that antibiotics have become "drugs of fear," so called by Dr. Calvin Kunin, chief of infectious diseases at Ohio State University School of Medicine. In this era of complex diseases and litigation, not only are physicians unsure of their diagnostic acumen and afraid they might miss a disease that could have been treated, which could lead to a bad outcome, perhaps even death, for their patient, but they are also afraid of being sued for not covering all the bases. Antibiotics have become a main weapon for practicing defensive medicine.

But it goes deeper than that. Physicians widely believe that there is virtually no downside to giving antibiotics, that they are perfectly safe to use under any circumstances. They don't understand that they are contributing to the development of resistance whenever they use this illogical approach. To paraphrase one of Bill Cosby's best routines, most of our doctors have flunked antibiotics.

In the United States we are more than thirty years removed from the days of the "dispensing physician" when doctors routinely sold drugs to patients out of their offices. And although physicians in this country have often been accused of not giving their patients enough information about what disease they have and just how it is being treated, it has never really been taken to the extremes that still exist in Japan, where doctors keep their patients in the dark as a matter of course, frequently concealing diagnoses and covering up the labels on pill bottles.

But physicians in the United States are still the ultimate filter through which all therapeutic decisions pass. Because we have entrusted them with that responsibility and authority, we have every right to expect that the decisions our physicians make will be based on a solid understanding of disease processes and the latest and most effective treatments for them. Unfortunately, this is often not the case.

The real trouble is with our medical education system, and the problems begin early. In the first two years of school, medical students learn a tremendous amount about the basic biological sciences, first how the healthy body functions when they study anatomy, biochemistry, physiology and histology, and then the mechanisms of disease when they study pathology and microbiology. They also study pharmacology, in which they are taught about the many classes of drugs to treat conditions such as cardiovascular disease, gastrointestinal problems and infections. But during the study of microbiology, the students are taught very little about antibiotic resistance and how it develops, and in the study of pharmacology they learn mostly about the biochemical mechanism of action of therapeutic drugs. This is certainly information important for doctors to know, but it isn't enough in the real world of treating patients. Knowledge doesn't always translate into know-how.

The logical time for medical students to learn how to apply to patient therapeutics the theoretical knowledge they have gained in their basic science training is in the final two years of medical school, when they spend most of their time in the hospital dealing with patients. But according to Dr. Jerry Avorn, professor of social medicine and health policy at Harvard Medical School, this sort of teaching is not undertaken nearly enough or in any organized way.

Instead, students pretty much muddle through these last two years, following in cookbook fashion what the senior resident does without learning the thinking process that should go into deciding when an antibiotic should be administered and when it shouldn't, what antibiotics are best to use in a variety of circumstances and how long a course of treatment should be.

This lack of the right kind of education continues after medical school, in the residency years and then into private practice. In fact, it is usually the case that the further removed a physician is from his basic medical training, the more uninformed he becomes. Inadequate though it may be, at least there is some formal training in the use of antibiotics during medical school and residency. But other than being left to their own devices, for practicing physicians there really is no official mechanism in place to ensure that they stay up to date. It may be reasonable to assume that doctors, intelligent, well paid, and for the most part dedicated, would and should take it upon themselves to keep abreast of the medical literature. But even with the best of intentions, most physicians fail to do that. The exigencies of running a busy practice, making daily hospital rounds and complying with an increasingly unwieldy and demanding administrative bureaucracy leave them little spare time to catch up on their medical journals. Perhaps we can commiserate with them, but we can't forgive them. The stakes are too high.

Because the Food and Drug Administration approves approximately twenty to thirty new drugs every year, within just ten years after doctors complete formal training, the entire pharmacopeia could be as foreign to those who don't keep up as it was on the first day they entered medical school. Not only are they unsure how to choose the appropriate drug, the drugs themselves are unfamiliar. This is especially true of antibiotics, because there so many of them are introduced every year. For example, since the first two cephalosporins were approved by the Food and Drug Administration in the mid-1960s, there has been an exponential increase in the different kinds of this type of antibiotic. Presently, there are three generations of cephalosporins (with a fourth generation on the immediate horizon) and more than twenty individual generic substances available for a doctor to choose from. Without a solid educational base as a guide, and with the names of most cephalosporins both tongue-twisters and so similar to one another, it's virtually impossible for physicians to keep up with advances in antibiotics unless they make a serious effort to do so.

The existence of this great educational void was recognized by pharmaceutical companies a long time ago, and naturally they saw it as a wide-open door of opportunity. They would be able to educate doctors about antibiotics and other drugs, putting their own spin on the process. In other words, they would teach physicians how, why and when to prescribe their products. The industry reasoned that the most effective way to do this would be to get hold of fledgling physicians when their medical minds were still malleable. Therefore, most of the major pharmaceutical firms establish strong ties with medical students as early in their training as possible. I still have on a bookshelf in my den the black doctor's bag traditionally given to students by a drug company on their first day of medical school. I had reason to be grateful to Lilly before I looked at my first histology slide through my newly purchased microscope or made my first cut on the cadaver in gross anatomy lab. And although Lilly has discontinued its black bag largess, it by no means is a sign that the pharmaceutical company–medical student liaison has been in any way weakened. The industry continues to find novel and creative ways of ingratiating itself with medical students.

Naturally, this relationship doesn't end after medical school. Like a fine Bordeaux, it gets deeper and better with age, through residency and into the practicing life of the physician. Once a doctor is in practice, the pharmaceutical industry spends an average of five thousand dollars per physician annually. The majority of this money is spent in the area of promotion or advertising, and a good bit of the promotion to doctors takes place in face-to-face meetings. Every day, salesmen from the pharmaceutical companies cool their heels in physicians' waiting rooms, sitting right among the patients and distinguished from them only by their large sample cases. Not all of them will be seen on a given day, but they make the best of even a brief audience. Dr. Avorn describes the process as follows:

"The companies make expert use of the most effective tools available in generating behavior change: person-to-person contact with practitioners through salespeople ('detailers') who make up in affability, small gifts and extensive knowledge of sales techniques what they lack in clinical expertise; the wide dissemination of visually arresting, persuasive and emotionally involving print materials; and frequent repetition of messages containing a few basic concepts. The more staid, visually unstimulating format of the medical literature itself, though replete with data, careful methodology and references, often fares poorly next to the effective marketing strategies that inevitably surround research findings."

Not surprisingly, several studies, including some conducted by Dr. Avorn, have shown that it is primarily from contact with pharmaceutical company representatives that physicians obtain most of their information about new drugs. On several levels, physicians like dealing with the drug company reps. It allows them to tell themselves they are keeping up with the latest developments when they prescribe the newest (and often most expensive) antibiotic on the market. Most physicians also have healthy egos and enjoy the practiced obsequiousness of the detailers. But doctors also know that they are not the most objective source of information. When interviewed, physicians naturally don't like to admit that this is the source of their knowledge; many are probably unaware of how much they rely on the pharmaceutical reps. And some of these detailers will frankly admit to being embarrassed at how easily they have been able to manipulate a doctor into prescribing their drug.

Besides direct contact with doctors through their sales reps, the pharmaceutical companies find other means of getting their message out. Open any issue of any medical journal and you'll find as many advertisements for drugs as you will plugs for moisturizers, clothes and jewelry in Vogue. And these ads are just as slickly produced, the print counterpart of a visit from a salesman.

If the net result of thousands of visits from thousands of detailers every day is an increased number of antibiotic prescriptions—and we can be certain that it is, or else the industry wouldn't continue to spend the billions on promotion every year that it does—it seems pretty convenient to throw a good deal of the blame for the inappropriate use of antibiotics on the pharmaceutical industry.

But how guilty are the drug companies? Not very, in the opinion of several of the most respected academicians in the United States, those whose ethics are beyond reproach. One of them is Dr. Avorn of Harvard, who has been most vocal about the deficiencies in medical education. "About all we can accuse the pharmaceutical industry of is being aggressive," Dr. Avorn says. "And their activities are so tightly controlled by the FDA it would be difficult for them to cross the line if they wanted to." Dr. Daniel Musher, chief of infectious diseases at Baylor University School of Medicine, who has frequently warned his academic colleagues about forging relationships with drug companies that are too tight, agrees. "The drug companies are not the corporate villains that they have been depicted to be," Dr. Musher says. "They're only doing what they're in business to do: sell a product."

And, we might add, a product that has already received approval from the Food and Drug Administration, meaning that in the FDA's eyes it is a product with genuine therapeutic merit. Unfortunately, this approval process has become more and more protracted and expensive over the years. To gain approval for a new drug, it usually takes a drug company twelve years and more than $230 million to jump through all the bureaucratic hoops. Since total patent protection is only seventeen years, the company generally has only five years to try and recoup its R & D investment and make a profit before the generic versions of the drug come along and eat up 50 percent of its market share within just a few years. Being acutely aware of the ticking clock undoubtedly increases the aggressive posture of the drug companies. Does the Food and Drug Administration have to share at least some of the criticism that has been directed at the pharmaceutical industry?

If so, drug companies cannot be let off the hook completely. Although objective analysis leads to the conclusion that they have been the victims of more bad press in the past few years than they rightfully deserve, much of it has been self-inflicted. Dr. Avorn and Dr. Musher may have been a little too kind.

In the golden age of antibiotics, from the late 1940s through the 1960s, the pharmaceutical companies were heroes. Time and again, they came up with miraculous inventions or discoveries, and not just in the area of antibiotics. Few of us have not been touched either directly or indirectly by their genius. But their reputation began to sour in the 1970s, when Senator Ted Kennedy turned the intense light of government scrutiny on the promotional activities of the pharmaceutical industry. The investigation led to the discovery of several campaigns that were at best unethical; some were perhaps illegal. And the wattage was cranked up even higher in December 1990 in a public and highly publicized hearing before a Senate committee, again chaired by Kennedy. For two days, a host of witnesses paraded before the committee and related their horror stories of inappropriate behavior by the drug companies. Although there were rebuttals from spokesmen for the industry, including Gerald Mossinghoff, who until 1993 was president of the Pharmaceutical Manufacturers Association, the organization that represents all the major pharmaceutical companies, they were largely drowned out by the accusations.

The chief hatchet man was Dr. Sidney Wolfe, president of the Washington, D.C.–based Public Citizen Health Research Group, a consumer activist organization. Dr. Wolfe, a brilliant and articulate physician, has long been waging war against what he considers illegal activities of the pharmaceutical industry. Among the specifics pointed out by Dr. Wolfe were a "frequent-flier/frequent-prescriber program," in which a physician would get frequent-flier miles on American Airlines every time he or she wrote a prescription for an antihypertensive drug; direct payments to physicians for using an antibiotic, offered under the guise of research but characterized by Dr. Wolfe as an out-and-out bribe; a free in-office computer system for physicians so that pharmaceutical companies would have access only to the medical records (with names of patients deleted), and therefore the prescribing practices, of a physician, and as part of the deal, a subscribing physician had to agree to a command performance and watch a set number of promotional messages each month. There were also a whole slew of examples of what Dr. Wolfe called "wining, dining and pocket-lining," in which physicians would either be taken on trips with their spouses to lavish tropical resorts or to the Super Bowl, or be merely given one hundred or two hundred dollars to attend dinner meetings at which a particular drug would be promoted.

It still remains a matter of interpretation as to whether all the charges leveled by Dr. Wolfe at the 1990 hearing were true. And even if they were, while certainly not excusing them, the general consensus has been that such practices are not institutionalized, but rather are the concoctions of overzealous marketing managers. But the accusations embarrassed the industry. A frequent-flier/frequent-prescriber program might win a creativity award from *Advertising Age* magazine but it's not going to score any points for integrity. Those in charge should have been more cognizant of how sensitive an industry they were in. Whenever companies profit from the misery and illness of others—even when those profits are justified—they are going to be vulnerable to criticism. They must take the high road.

The upshot of this negative publicity was the formulation of a code of ethics by both the American Medical Association and the Pharmaceutical Manufacturers Association, which was later adopted and put into law by the Food and Drug Administration. In essence, this code does two things. It clearly delineates the promotional activities and the educational activities of drug companies. Anything that falls within the promotional category need not be what the FDA calls "fair and balanced." While obviously prohibited from lying, drug companies, either in face-to-face visits or in print advertising, are under no obligation to tell a doctor about how another product stacks up against theirs—and are unlikely to do so unless, of course, it makes their drug look better. If an activity is delineated by the drug company as educational rather than promotional (more about educational activities shortly), the rules are changed. And the most basic difference is that any information delineated as educational *is* required to be "fair and balanced." It has to take on the character of a medical school lecture or a paper in a scientific journal.

The other thing the code does is limit the type of gifts that can be given by drug companies. Even if the activity is strictly promotional, no longer are expensive vacations allowed. Nor can doctors be given cash payments for attending dinner meetings promoting a drug. They are allowed to receive modest gifts, but they have to be medically related, such as a textbook, and chosen from an FDA-approved catalogue.

The enactment of a specific code of ethics did not, however, wipe the bull's-eye off the back of the pharmaceutical industry. In 1992, for example, a study was published in the *Annals of Internal Medicine* that evaluated how accurate drug company advertisements in medical journals were. Since these ads are a major source of information about pharmaceuticals for doctors, just what they contained is of obvious importance. The authors of the study from UCLA Medical School concluded that more than one-third of all drug company advertisements in scientific journals contained material that was misleading, especially in regard to efficacy and the conditions for which that drug should be used.

The study has since come under a great deal of criticism, primarily by Dr. Jacob Jacoby of New York University School of Medicine, a respected scientist in this area who has been a major contributor to the FDA guidelines as to what constitutes misleading advertising and who, in fact, was quoted in the study. Researchers at the Wharton School of Business were also critical of the statistical methods and concluded that, based on this study, no conclusions could be drawn. But while the original UCLA paper was widely publicized on television and in the most influential newspapers, including *The New York Times* and *The Wall Street Journal*, the refutations were hardly noticed. The bad taste in the public's mouth about drug company advertising lingers.

Even if some of the pharmaceutical company advertisements were determined to be misleading, isn't there some hypocrisy at work here as well? Shouldn't those who publish the advertisements be open to criticism? In the very same issue of the *Annals of Internal Medicine* in which this critical study appeared, there were dozens of pages of the same type of ads that the study was criticizing. It happens in all the medical journals. The editors of many of them have frequently taken an ivory tower position in relation to pharmaceutical promotions but have accepted the ads anyway. Their excuse: while the articles in the journals are peer-reviewed for accuracy, the ads are not and the physician should realize that. Translation: we couldn't publish our journal without the pharmaceutical money these advertisements bring.

Promotion and advertising aside, there's a more basic bone we've got to pick with drug companies, more sins of omission than of commission. First of all, how could they not foresee the massive problem of antibiotic resistance? Just as they haven't believed all the bad press they've received in the past few years, they shouldn't have believed all the plaudits directed their way when they kept coming up with one effective antibiotic after another. And if they did see that bacteria are gaining on us, they could have been doing something about it. Pharmaceutical scientists could have begun to concentrate their ingenuity, not on more "me-too antibiotics," drugs whose mechanism of action is not unique, but on researching new and better ways of subduing bacteria, methods that wouldn't perpetuate the resistance problem. And there could have been better communication between the scientific arms of these mammoth companies and their marketing arms. Drug company salesmen can't be expected to help educate physicians about antibiotic resistance if they aren't taught about it by the pharmaceutical researchers in the first place.

It would be naive to assume we've seen the last of promotional campaigns for drugs that cross the "responsible" line. Some ambitious product manager at some company will still think that the best way to move up the corporate ladder is to do whatever it takes to sell the product, and ethics be damned. But the pharmaceutical industry is not anxious for another volley of negative publicity, so it's likely that it really will police itself tightly, and violations of the code, in spirit or in letter, will become more and more anomalous.

Of course, just because drug company advertising and promotion will probably walk the straight and narrow doesn't mean the message is going to be any different, only the vehicle for its delivery. Physicians who rely exclusively or primarily on pharmaceutical promotions for their information are still going to be getting a highly biased message. So the focus returns to the doctors. Those getting the majority of their education from encounters with pharmaceutical detailers or advertisements in medical journals may not be participating in something illegal or even unethical, but they can be accused of intellectual laziness. And where our health is at stake—in the case of the unnecessary use of antibiotics, it's the health of all of us—this is a sin only slightly less reprehensible. Physicians aren't naive about the type of message the pharmaceutical companies deliver. How about giving up an afternoon of golf and reading the medical journals?

And in whatever unethical and illegal promotional campaigns have been conducted, doctors also have to shoulder a good portion of the blame. American Airlines stated in the 1990 hearing that its frequent-flier/frequent-prescriber program was one of the most successful campaigns it had ever been involved with. No one drafted all those doctors aboard. In order for the physicians' ethics to be corrupted, they had to be willing participants. Hippocrates must have turned over in his grave.

There is another area in which physicians deserve criticism. Over the last decade and a half, there has evolved a mechanism that has the potential to compete with the unbalanced messages of pharmaceutical promotion: Continuing Medical Education. CME programs have become increasingly popular, as more and more specialty boards have instituted requirements that physicians attend a certain number of approved courses and obtain a requisite number of CME credits each year. Sounds like the answer, doesn't it? As of now, however, CME remains a potential, because not enough doctors have taken advantage of the opportunities.

"The way Continuing Medical Education has been handled is nothing less than a travesty," Dr. Avorn says. There are a few reasons for this. First, there simply haven't been enough good courses available. Those that are offered and qualify as relevant and objective are usually given under the auspices of an academic institution, such as Harvard Medical School or the Mayo Clinic. But the presence of these courses in a catalogue, or even the presence of physicians at the course itself, is no guarantee that they actually learn any new information. In order for doctors to be handed the CME certificate that they then send in to their specialty board as proof they participated in the course, all they have to do is log in at the conference. No one ever checks to see if the doctor snoozed through the seminar discussing the pros and cons of a new antibiotic, or if he was even there at all. Once he has signed in, he can spend the rest of the time at Disney World with his family, and no one will be the wiser.

I can personally vouch for this happening. When I was a practicing pathologist, I generally attended two or three such meetings a year. At one of them, a January conference on forensic medicine in

Snowbird, Utah, during ski season, I knew of a colleague who spent far more time on the slopes than he did in the sessions. Yet along with his tan and improved slalom technique, he received the same official-looking CME certificate as those of us who attended all the sessions.

There has been of late, however, some evidence that the CME system may be improving. Help is coming from what many would consider not only an unlikely but an untrustworthy source: the pharmaceutical industry. The increased pharmaceutical industry presence in continuing education is expanding the number of courses available. And the way in which many of these courses are being implemented is making it more difficult for physicians to obtain certification without demonstrating they actually learned something.

We shouldn't assume, of course, that the pharmaceutical companies don't have as their ultimate motive the shedding of some attractive light on their products. But the messages delivered in CME courses in which they are involved are still going to be of great benefit. The code promulgated in 1990 requires it. The rules here are distinctly different from what is allowed in a purely promotional activity. The Food and Drug Administration is aware that the tenuous alliance between doctors and drug companies could easily become an unholy one and has therefore instituted tight regulations to ensure things stay on the up and up.

Although a few pharmaceutical companies have in-house Continuing Medical Education departments to produce courses for physicians, the Food and Drug Administration has increasingly frowned on this setup as far too incestuous; in fact, it is about to become illegal. What is becoming the standard is for a pharmaceutical company to give an outright grant to an academic institution desirous of presenting a Continuing Medical Education program. The institution, either through its own staff or by working with an outside independent facilitator, then devises the entire program, including not only the logistics, such as where it will be held, in conjunction with what national meeting, at what hotel, etc., but also the specific topics to be discussed.

The pharmaceutical companies that confer the educational grants are allowed to have input of only two types. They are allowed to know in advance of donating the funds what general topic the academic institution is interested in presenting. Will it be on infectious disease or hypertension or Alzheimer's disease? And if it is about infection, will it be urinary infections, AIDS or bronchitis? If a pharmaceutical company has recently introduced a new antibiotic for the treatment of pneumonia, it would be primarily interested in funding an educational meeting where physicians learn about the latest advances in lower respiratory tract infections, the hope being, of course, that more doctors will use the new antibiotic. Knowing the general subject, pharmaceutical companies are also allowed to make recommendations to either the academic institution or the facilitator about who are the opinion leaders in the field. The Food and Drug Administration recognizes that the pharmaceutical company is probably in the best position to identify these scientists because they have spent a great deal of money sponsoring research on drugs in that field. But it is also recognized that those recommended are likely to be favorably inclined toward the sponsoring company's product, so in no way is the CME provider obligated to follow its recommendations.

Beyond that, the pharmaceutical company providing the educational grant is required to keep hands off. In fact, the FDA is so concerned that the funding company not exert any further influence on the content of the continuing education program, either directly or indirectly (e.g., if the academic institution believes that future financial support for research projects and other activities may depend on its producing programs that somehow promote the company's products), that it insists on a written agreement stating the independence of the provider from the influence of the supporting company. This makes it highly likely that the material presented at one of these courses will comply with the FDA requirement that it be "fair and balanced."

As a further safeguard, neither the academic institution nor the grant-providing pharmaceutical company is allowed to pick up any expenses for the presenters at a course, other than modest travel and lodging and a small honorarium. And, breaking with past traditions, it is forbidden to pick up the tab at all for any physicians who merely attend the program. They must all pay their own travel, lodging and registration fees.

Marketing managers at most of the pharmaceutical companies can be extremely creative, so they will be continuing to look for loopholes where they can somehow promote their products but stay within the increasingly rigid legal and ethical guidelines. And occasionally they may succeed. On balance, however, the messages delivered by these programs are going to be largely educational.

Those who are critical of the drug companies participating in Continuing Medical Education courses should realize a basic fact: they are quite expensive to produce, and if the pharmaceutical industry were removed from the CME scene, there would be far fewer of these courses available. Isn't it far better to have an abundance of these courses available, and count on the physicians to discern any bias in favor of a drug company's products?

Many of these pharmaceutical-company-sponsored courses are also beginning to address the basic educational deficiency and include tests that the participants must pass before being awarded their CME certificate. At present most of the tests are too easy. A physician attendee could still spend much of his time snorkeling and probably get the CME credits. But it's a step in the right direction. Now it's up to the doctors to take advantage of these opportunities.

Finally, we must point the finger at one other group: ourselves. Although the recommendation of drugs is supposed to be the physician's purview, that's not always the way it works. Patients often put pressure on their doctors and demand prescriptions, sometimes even stipulating the brand name desired. This is frequently the scenario when a doctor gives a patient an antibiotic for a cold. Every physician has had this experience. Just the other day, I had a call from a relative who described the symptoms of a viral illness and practically begged me to call in a prescription for an antibiotic. When I refused, she angrily hung up on me.

When a doctor's practice is at stake, however, the resolution is often different. Especially in large cities, physicians are experiencing more and more competition for patients. If a doctor doesn't end the visit for a viral illness with the asked-for prescription for an antibiotic, his patient is likely to go down the street to another doctor who will comply. The patient will then become a former patient.

What it really comes down to, then, is that there are few segments of our society that can escape some measure of blame for inappropriate antibiotic use. And when we talk about solutions, we must address all of them.

CHAPTER 11

Fifteen Things You Can Do to Avert Catastrophe

Given the perils of the inappropriate use of antibiotics, it is a practice that must be stopped. And all of us can play a part in the following program. This is not a program for you to read and set aside. It is a call to action—your action. In virtually every one of the facets of this plan, there is something you can do. In some cases, you can apply the advice to yourself. But most of the time you will be called upon to interact with either your physician, a medical society or the government. The specific names and addresses of those you should contact appear in the last section of this book. Implementing the plan will cost money from funding authorities, so we all must be insistent and persistent. We can no longer ignore the problem. The stakes are too high.

1. MEDICAL STUDENTS AND RESIDENTS MUST BE TAUGHT WHAT THEY NEED TO KNOW ABOUT ANTIBIOTICS

Dr. Donald Kollisch is a family practitioner who has been on both sides of the fence, formerly in private practice and now as a teacher in the family practice residency program at the University of North

Carolina School of Medicine. He admitted to me that he was appalled at how little his colleagues or the students and residents who pass through his service know about the clinical use of antibiotics. "The time has come to stop giving students lists of germs to memorize in microbiology and integrate it more with clinical teaching," he said. "It is the only way we can prepare them for dealing with patients."

Dr. Kollisch suggests that in the first two years of medical school—the so-called preclinical years when students spend most of their time in classrooms or laboratories—during microbiology classes, whenever the structure and physiology of a particular type of bacterium are being taught, the students should be taken to the hospital floor to observe a patient infected with that organism. If the topic of the lecture that day is *Streptococcus pneumoniae,* then a patient with the pneumonia it causes should be examined. Right then and there a discussion should be held about how best to treat that patient, which antibiotic to use and why, and it should be correlated with strong admonitions about inappropriate use and the development of resistance. Only then will the integrated message hit home. "If the same plan is carried forward into residency, perhaps we can start turning out doctors who understand more how to deal with the resistance problem," Dr. Kollisch said.

What you can do: Strongly urge your physician to put pressure on specialty board organizations, local and state medical societies, and the American Medical Association; also include the American Association of Medical Colleges and the Liaison Committee on Medical Education, the two organizations that oversee the standardized medical school curriculum taught in the United States. Regardless of whether your doctor agrees or not, write to these organizations. Encourage everyone you know to do the same.

2. PHYSICIANS MUST TAKE PERIODIC RECERTIFICATION EXAMS IN WHICH THEY ARE TESTED ON ANTIBIOTIC KNOWLEDGE IN ORDER TO RETAIN THEIR MEDICAL LICENSE

The increasing number of Continuing Medical Education courses that are becoming available is a good start. But it's not nearly enough. First, it must be made mandatory for every physician who is in the position of prescribing or monitoring antibiotics (we could exempt, for example, psychiatrists, radiologists and physiatrists—specialists in physical medicine and rehabilitation) to take an annual update course in antibiotics and infectious diseases, with emphasis on appropriate usage to avoid selection for resistant strains of bacteria. Second, every few years it would be required for physicians to pass an exam on this knowledge, not only in order to remain in good standing with one's specialty board but also to retain the license to practice medicine. This could, and should, include knowledge in other areas of medicine as well, but antibiotics cut across all specialty lines and are the key component.

There is a bit of good news here. As a bold first step, the American Board of Family Practice has already begun recertifying its member physicians and there is talk that the American Board of Internal Medicine will do the same. What we need now is to extend recertification to surgeons, obstetrician-gynecologists and pediatricians, make certain the material the doctors are being tested on includes the right information about antibiotics, and tie it in to license renewal.

What you can do: Lobbying your physician for recertification is likely to fall upon deaf, perhaps even hostile, ears. While intellectually admitting the desirability or even the necessity of periodic recertification, few doctors would relish having to study as they did in medical school. But thousands of calls and letters to the state medical boards that control doctors' licenses, as well as to the various specialty boards, can be a strong incentive for change. Ask your congressional representatives and senators (both state and federal) to intervene and put further pressure on the licensing boards.

3. GIVE HOSPITAL PHARMACISTS VETO POWER OVER DOCTORS

As so many antibiotic-resistant bacteria are bred in hospitals, a great deal of effort must be concentrated there. Strong reins must be put on profligate prescribing of antibiotics.

Some small inroads have already been made in this area. According to both Dr. Calvin Kunin, chief of infectious diseases at Ohio State University School of Medicine and the physician responsible for establishing the antibiotic auditing system used in most hospitals, and Dr. Harry Gallis, an infectious disease specialist at Duke University Medical School, there has recently been improvement in the way prophylactic antibiotics are administered by surgeons. The short course is beginning to catch on. As approximately half the antibiotics used in hospitals are for prophylactic purposes, the pressure to limit antibiotics for this use to only one dose before surgery needs to be continued.

The way to make certain that occurs, as well as improving other areas of antibiotic use in hospitals, is to put restrictions on the antibiotics physicians can use and the situations in which they can use them. In this scenario, the hospital pharmacist is someone you may be able to trust more than your own doctor to make intelligent decisions about antibiotics. The pharmacist occupies an influential position on the hospital formulary committee, the organization in the hospital that determines what are the appropriate antibiotics to treat certain conditions. The pharmacist doesn't act alone on the committee—there are usually infectious disease specialists, infection control nurses and the hospital administrator as well—but the burden of assessing and sometimes vetoing doctors' orders falls on him. What will keep the members of such committees pure, free of pressure from the pharmaceutical companies lobbying to have their antibiotics kept off the restricted list, is going to be the increased emphasis on managed care. To hold down costs, there will be more significance placed on both using the cheaper antibiotics and using them for only the length of time and in the situations for which they are needed. As an upshot of these money-saving policies, the emergence of resistant strains will be held in check.

Mandatory restrictions have already been tried in some institutions with varying degrees of success. Dr. Stephen Barriere is a hospital pharmacist at UCLA Medical Center (like many hospital pharmacists he has an advanced degree called a Pharm.D.) who chairs the formulary committee. Dr. Barriere told me that things in his institution have worked out pretty well. Because repeated audits revealed overuse, restrictions were placed on the administration of several newer and more expensive antibiotics, including ciprofloxacin, imipenem and the combination drug ampicillin/sulbactam. Every time a physician orders one of these drugs at UCLA there has to be a "mandatory consult" with the pharmacy department to determine whether the order is justified. If in the view of Dr. Barriere the antibiotic is not justified, he has the authority to veto the order and ask the doctor to prescribe another antibiotic. As might be expected, Dr. Barriere told me that physicians first bristled at having their authority questioned in this manner, but eventually came to accept that if they learned the appropriate circumstances for prescribing the drugs on the restricted list, their orders would be approved.

But Dr. Barriere and other formulary committees also found out that the guard can never be relaxed. According to Dr. Cheryl Himmelberg, also a Pharm.D. at the University of North Carolina School of Medicine, while the mandatory consult/veto program was in place at her hospital, inappropriate antibiotic use and bacterial resistance declined. As soon as the restrictions were lifted, however, it was like floodgates breaking, and the number of prescriptions for the previously restricted drugs increased by 158 percent. Clearly, these restrictions need to be kept in place, and not only in just a few teaching hospitals around the country, but in every hospital where a formulary committee exists.

What you can do: Once again, for obvious reasons, your doctor is not the best conduit to action. Put pressure on the administrators of hospitals in your area. Write to the Joint Commission on the Accreditation of Healthcare Organizations and insist that mandatory restrictions be placed on antibiotic ordering.

4. EDUCATE PHYSICIANS VIA COMPUTER AT THE TIME THEY ORDER AN ANTIBIOTIC

Dr. Jerry Avorn, professor of social medicine and health policy at Harvard Medical School, is a pioneer in the field of physicians' prescribing habits and how to change them. Although he is not against the hospital pharmacist having veto power, he believes that physicians may respond just as well to a softer sell, a more educational approach. In some cases, such as the larger hospitals where there is a formulary committee, the two methods could be tried in tandem.

One plan Dr. Avorn recommends is a consultation, not with the hospital pharmacist, but with the infectious disease specialist. This meeting would also be mandatory, but the difference is that no veto power would be involved. Instead of restricting a doctor from using a particular antibiotic, the infectious disease specialist would try to educate his fellow physician about why antibiotic X may be a better choice to reduce propagation of resistance than antibiotic Y. Dr. Avorn is confident that most doctors under these circumstances will make the correct choice and won't need shackles. This procedure has been tested in only a limited manner, however, and the soft sell clearly needs more trials. The veto should loom in the background, ready to be called into action if necessary.

Dr. Avorn has also developed a more innovative educational approach, operating on the same foundation that doctors will make the appropriate decisions if presented with the correct information at the right time. To that end, he has created the structured educational order form for antibiotics. For the program to work, it is mandatory that hospital policy be changed so that any antibiotic ordered must be entered on the structured form, different for each antibiotic. The form contains educational messages and graphic reminders about the proper use of the antibiotic being ordered, not only what infections it should be used for—for example, "the aminoglycoside antibiotic of choice in this hospital is gentamicin unless infection with *Pseudomonas* is suspected or proven"—but also the recommended dose and length of administration. The message is very similar to the highly effective pharmaceutical advertisements that physicians read in their medical journals, colorful and eye-catching.

Dr. Avorn designed this form in 1988, and in limited testing it has worked very well to bring physicians' antibiotic prescribing habits into line. In one study he conducted, the use of the most expensive antibiotics (the same ones that are newest and to which it is vital to preserve bacterial sensitivity) plummeted by more than 70 percent.

A very attractive feature of the structured order form is that Dr. Avorn is already adapting it to be used on computers, the vehicle by which most antibiotics will be ordered by the end of the decade. "This will provide an even greater opportunity to educate hospital staff physicians," Dr. Avorn told me. The software he is developing not only will be able to keep up to date with the antibiotic sensitivity patterns in the hospital and feed them back to the physician at the time the antibiotic is ordered on the computer terminal, but will be interactive as well. It will provide an individualized tutorial about the prescribing of the particular antibiotic, right at the time the order is being placed, the time when the doctor will be most receptive to being educated.

In addition, this computerized order form/tutorial is easily exportable. Of the more than eight thousand hospitals in the United States, over half of them are community hospitals with fewer than one hundred beds. Few of these smaller hospitals have the personnel for a well-structured formulary committee (infectious disease specialists, for example, in these settings are almost nonexistent). But they all have personal computers. If Dr. Avorn's software is installed, it will provide the equivalent of a private consultation with an infectious disease expert every time an antibiotic is ordered.

What you can do: Write to the Joint Commission on the Accreditation of Healthcare Organizations and ask that Dr. Avorn's program, or one similar to it, be made mandatory. Talk to your local hospital administrator, especially in the community hospitals.

5. INSTALL HIGH-TECH HAND-WASHERS IN HOSPITALS

The introduction of disposable latex gloves several decades ago was an inestimable contribution to medicine. But there has been a backlash. More than one expert observer has reported that the ability to pull gloves on and off at will has made hospital personnel far too complacent about a most basic principle of infection control: hand-washing. We have forgotten the principles of Semmelweis.

Just as we described earlier, in the story of the *Serratia-Klebsiella* multihospital Nashville epidemic in the 1970s, most nosocomial infections are transmitted on the hands of health care workers. Pathogenic gram-negative bacteria can survive on the hands for over two hours, as can others, including the very dangerous methicillin-resistant staph bacteria.

In a meticulous study conducted for more than eight months, involving almost two thousand patients and reported in 1992 in the *New England Journal of Medicine,* Dr. Richard Wenzel and his colleagues at the University of Iowa College of Medicine found that not only did more frequent and thorough hand-washing by hospital personnel significantly reduce the transmission of infections, but what was used as a washing agent was important as well. Many hospitals use a combination of rubbing alcohol and soap, which proved not nearly as effective in reducing the nosocomial infection rate as the antimicrobial disinfectant chlorhexidine.

An innovative means of dispensing chlorhexidine could be a high-tech hand-washer—a small unit with two round openings in which a photocell activates spinning jets of the antibacterial solution. Limited studies have shown it cleanses even more thoroughly than standard washing procedure and that people are more likely to use it than other methods.

What you can do: Again, write to the Joint Commission on the Accreditation of Healthcare Organizations and visit your local hospital administrator. Insist that a strictly enforced hand-washing policy be instituted, preferably employing a high-tech hand-washer, which can be purchased for about six thousand dollars, a small price to pay if it will encourage more frequent washing and reduce transmission of resistant bacteria.

6. BALANCE THE PHARMACEUTICAL SALES PITCH

Programs need to be put in place to address inappropriate prescribing by office-based physicians as well; much of this is the result of doctors relying too heavily on pharmaceutical detailers for their information. Dr. Avorn has also devised a solution here. "Let the sales reps come in and take their best shot," he said, "but at the same time, let's put some mechanisms in place to strike a balance."

The impetus for this is proving to be not antibiotic resistance but money, but if applied correctly the result will be the same. Many of the large, powerful corporations in the United States are turning to managed health care for their employees and in so doing have determined that many of the antibiotic prescriptions written are unnecessary expenses. In order to address this, several managed care companies now employ specially trained pharmacists whose sole function is to visit physicians and counterbalance the sales pitch they receive from the pharmaceutical industry.

This program has been called counterdetailing, but Dr. Avorn prefers the term academic detailing. A session might go like this: A detailing pharmacist says, "I know you've heard a lot about Cipro, Doctor, and it's a good drug, but did you know that in an otherwise healthy woman with a urinary tract infection caused by *E. coli,* ampicillin is still the antibiotic of choice?" Controlled studies by Dr. Avorn and Dr. William Schaffner of Vanderbilt University indicated that academic detailing could be quite successful in bringing doctors' antibiotic prescribing patterns into line.

The large Kaiser Program in California has already adopted academic detailing, and according to Don Kitajima of Kaiser Northern California in Oakland, the pharmacist at the helm, early results are encouraging. Medco, a large drug-benefits manager in Montvale, New Jersey, has been employed by Blue Cross and Blue Shield of Massachusetts (Dr. Avorn is their chief consultant) to do the same thing. The Veterans Administration is also considering adopting academic detailing.

What you can do: If you belong to an HMO or other managed care organization, ask if it is using a similar program. If not, explain to the administrator why it should be and put him in touch with either Don

Kitajima at Kaiser in San Francisco or Terry Latanich at Medco to get the particulars of the academic detailing program and how the hospital can become involved.

7. ENCOURAGE USE OF A COMPUTER PROGRAM FOR DOCTORS' OFFICES THAT HELPS THEM PRESCRIBE ANTIBIOTICS APPROPRIATELY

To reinforce the academic detailing, an instrument is needed for physicians' offices such as we advocated for hospitals, a computer program that provides feedback to the doctor at the time of getting ready to write a prescription for an antibiotic. It wouldn't have the mandatory aspect of the hospital-based system, but the desire for good information and the pressure of periodic antibiotic audits by the state or county medical societies would provide incentive for the physician to use the software.

There is already one such program available called Antibiotica PC: Infectious Disease Analytical Software, available from a small company called MacroMed in Whittier, California. I purchased a copy of this program, and although it has some flaws, it is still valuable for a physician to have. Undoubtedly there will be other programs available soon. Dr. Avorn, for example, is working on an office version of his structured order form.

What you can do: Suggest to your physician that he or she purchase a copy of the software. The basic version is only one hundred dollars, the deluxe edition two hundred.

8. GIVE PATIENTS LIFE-STYLE PRESCRIPTIONS

Several surveys have been conducted which have shown that the majority of people still don't know the difference between a viral and a bacterial infection, and that antibiotics are effective only for the latter. Because of this lack of knowledge, many patients practically demand antibiotic prescriptions from their doctors for colds and other viral infections. As the writing of a prescription has become so inculcated into the modern office visit, rather than have physicians flatly refuse to offer a prescription when the situation is inappropriate, Dr. Avorn has come up with yet another vehicle, one that turns the act of prescription writing into a positive.

His idea is to give patients what looks just like a prescription but which, instead of providing an antibiotic, is a "life-style prescription," which carries an explanation of the difference between viral and bacterial infections, why antibiotics don't kill viruses and what the patients can do for their problem other than taking an antibiotic. "A prescription is a powerful sociological tool," says Dr. Avorn, "and this life-style prescription imbues the nonuse of drugs with the same clout as using them."

Life-style prescriptions can also be used on the other end of the spectrum. As many patients fail to finish their antibiotic prescriptions even where they are appropriately prescribed—a good situation for promoting growth of resistant bacteria—along with the antibiotic prescription could come a life-style prescription explaining the importance (with regard to resistance) of taking the entire dose.

What you can do: Besides never asking for an antibiotic prescription when it is not indicated and always finishing the ones you do get, encourage your doctor to contact Dr. Avorn at Harvard for more information about life-style prescriptions. Your physician should welcome this suggestion, as it could help relieve some of the unrelenting patient pressure to provide unnecessary antibiotics.

9. ENCOURAGE PHYSICIANS TO JOIN THE ALLIANCE FOR PRUDENT USE OF ANTIBIOTICS

The Alliance for Prudent Use of Antibiotics (APUA) was formed in 1981 by Dr. Stuart Levy, professor of microbiology and molecular biology at Tufts University Medical School and one of the world's recognized authorities on antibiotic abuse and bacterial resistance. It grew out of an international conference in the Dominican Republic that year, when Dr. Levy and more than one hundred fifty research scientists and clinicians signed an "Antibiotic Misuse

Statement." It was endorsed by health authorities worldwide, translated into many languages and featured in *Newsweek, Time, The New York Times* and *The Washington Post*. In the past decade, APUA has been communicating the basic tenets of proper antibiotic usage and highlighting areas of abuse around the world in a quarterly newsletter. As Dr. Levy says, "It is the only organization of its kind, dedicated solely to the improved use and knowledge about a therapeutic product, not a disease." Besides the newsletter, APUA is developing audiovisual programs for the general public as well as the medical profession.

What you can do: This is an excellent organization which has been severely underpublicized and underutilized. You can either join it yourself (the articles are not highly technical, less so, for example, than those in *Scientific American*) or at least encourage your doctor to join. If you are so inclined, you could give him or her a gift membership. There are various levels of membership (student to lifetime), and you can get one for less than fifty dollars. Even better, as APUA is designated a 501c3 corporation, the entire membership fee is tax-deductible.

10. SUPPORT A PROGRAM THAT LINKS ANTIBIOTIC RESISTANCE IN EVERY HOSPITAL IN THE WORLD

A vice president and member of the board of directors of APUA is Dr. Thomas O'Brien, the medical director of the microbiology laboratory at Brigham and Women's Hospital in Boston and an associate professor of medicine at Harvard Medical School. Dr. O'Brien strongly believes that a key ingredient in controlling the outbreak of antibiotic resistance is to recognize it quickly enough so that the appropriate controls can be put in place. Antibiotic-resistant bacteria can develop in Malaysia and rapidly find their way to Minneapolis or anywhere else in the world. If we knew that there had been an outbreak of resistance in Malaysia, we would be in a far better position to deal with it. "As the world's bacteria form networks to spread resistance to antibiotics, we need to build our own network to control that resistance," Dr. O'Brien told me.

To that end, Dr. O'Brien and his colleague Dr. John Stelling have developed an elegant piece of computer software that can take advantage of the fact that in every hospital in the world, even in developing countries, antibiotic sensitivity tests are done every day as a matter of course. The only additional step necessary would be to record the results of these tests on Dr. O'Brien's software, which he calls WHONET (the original funding came from the World Health Organization). A central computer in Boston would then be able to monitor resistance patterns throughout the world on a daily basis.

What you can do: There are forty thousand labs in the world that perform daily antibiotic sensitivity tests. WHONET is presently in only seventy of them. Expanding the program will take a couple of million dollars, small change in the larger scheme of things and an investment that will pay huge dividends. Unfortunately, the World Health Organization has contributed only five thousand dollars. Write WHO in Geneva, Switzerland, and urge it to free up money for this purpose. Write to Dr. Phillip Lee, the assistant secretary for Health and Human Services. Dr. Lee, whom we referred to earlier, is from the University of California, San Francisco, and has had a lifelong interest in the inappropriate use of antibiotics, especially in the developing world. The request for his support should fall on sympathetic ears.

Write to and call your senators and representatives asking for the same. Write to Vice President Al Gore, who in 1984 chaired a House Subcommittee Hearing on Antibiotic Resistance; at least he is aware of the dangers. In addition to money, there should be better cooperation from the governments in developing countries, where these resistant strains often arise, to import at least some of the newer antibiotics so that resistant infections aren't treated with old antibiotics, making the problem worse. Urge Vice President Gore and your congressional representatives to get involved in this area as well.

164 THE PLAGUE MAKERS

11. END THE USE OF ANTIBIOTICS AS GROWTH PROMOTERS IN ANIMALS

Although this is an issue that is still shrouded in controversy, special-interest lobbying and government bureaucracy, there is evidence that things are finally moving in the direction of eliminating, or at least drastically reducing the routine use of antibiotics in animals. But pressure must continue to be applied and from several directions.

What you can do: Make a donation to the Food Animal Concerns Trust (FACT) in Chicago, a privately financed, not-for-profit organization that supports farms where animals are raised without antibiotics added to their feed (this is also a 501c3 corporation, and your donation is tax-deductible). Encourage others to donate as well. Ask for products produced in this manner at your local supermarket and write its corporate headquarters. Nest Eggs, from chickens not fed antibiotics, are one example of such a product. With just one request, I convinced my local supermarket to carry them.

Put some pressure on the veterinary profession. If possible, begin at the grass-roots level and enlist the aid of your own veterinarian (if you use one) to contact the American Veterinary Association, urging it to issue an official statement deploring the wholesale use of sub-therapeutic doses of antibiotics in animals and supporting nonantibiotic growth promoters.

Contact the National Cattlemen's Association and the Poultry Science Association. Commend them for already advocating the elimination of penicillin and tetracycline from feed, and urge them to continue reminding farmers and livestock ranchers that there are alternatives such as monensin, a chemical used only for animals, and bacitracin and bambermycin, nonabsorbable antibiotics. Contact the National Pork Producers Council, which has done nothing thus far, and push it to follow the example of the others.

Contact the Natural Resources Defense Council in New York, an advocacy group of scientists and attorneys who have been pushing for a federal ban on antibiotics in animal feed for a decade. Ask what you can do to help advance their cause.

12. USE IMPROVED DIAGNOSTIC TESTS IN DOCTORS' OFFICES AND HOSPITALS

One of the main reasons why physicians use so much shotgun anti-biotic therapy is that they don't know what bacteria are causing an infection, or even if the infection is bacterial at all. In order for all the antibiotic software programs to be effective in directing doctors to-ward the appropriate narrow-spectrum drugs, first there must be quick and accurate means of identifying the organisms.

In this regard, hospital microbiology laboratories have improved a great deal in recent years, with most of their identification and sen-sitivity testing being done on fully automated instruments. But there is room for improvement. Physicians can start by making some of the diagnoses themselves. There are now several inexpensive kits available for in-office use that allow identification of *Streptococcus* from a throat swab or the offending bacteria from a urine specimen in less than twenty-four hours. In these cases, guessing about what organism is the cause of the infection is no longer necessary.

These kits, while valuable now, are merely interim steps to what's coming in rapid diagnosis. Segments of it are already available in some of the larger hospitals, will soon be available for community hospitals and within five years will be standard in most doctors' of-fices. We are talking about DNA probes, another outgrowth of the molecular biology revolution that is transforming medicine. Not only will these probes be able to identify bacteria from body fluids and tissues much more quickly than even the most sophisticated laboratory equipment now available—in many cases within just a few hours—but they will also be able to determine the antibiotic-resistance pattern of the bacteria.

The DNA probes are tiny pieces of genetic material that bind like molecular Velcro to complementary DNA fragments in a bacterial cell. Since each type of bacteria has its specific DNA, a probe will bind to a stretch of DNA that belongs to that type of organism ex-clusively. The DNA probe of a particular organism, for example, pneumococcus, will not bind to the DNA of staph. The probes are added to the specimen for identification, such as blood, feces, or urine, and within just a few hours analyzed to determine which bac-teria are present. By first subjecting the specimen to amplification with another novel technique called the polymerase chain reaction, or PCR (the same PCR is being used to identify human genes), which can increase the size of the sample by more than a billionfold, it is possible to identify the organism *from just a single cell*.

Once that has been accomplished, a second series of probes, designed to detect the DNA sequences of antibiotic-resistance genes rather than the entire organism, can be added. The applicability of this aspect of the test will depend on the availability of the corresponding DNA probes. Although several have been developed, many more are needed. As DNA probe technology becomes cheaper and more widely used, it could be not only available for the large teaching hospitals but routinely used in community hospitals and eventually in physicians' offices. Knowing precisely what they are dealing with in a matter of a few hours will provide the opportunity to cut down shotgun therapy dramatically.

What you can do: Ask your doctor if he uses the in-office diagnostic kits. Check with the hospitals in your area to see if the DNA probes are being tried, and if not, encourage their use. Write to the NIH and support research on DNA probe development.

13. MAKE BETTER USE OF EXISTING VACCINES

The better we can become at defeating bacterial invaders with our endogenous or internal capabilities, the less need there will be to use antibiotics. At the forefront in this area are vaccines, especially valuable for the elderly and the very young, the two groups whose immune systems are the least robust and therefore most vulnerable to infection.

This is especially true for pneumococcal pneumonia, which remains an important cause of morbidity and mortality among the elderly. According to Dr. David Fedson of the University of Virginia School of Medicine, as many as 120,000 adults over sixty-five are hospitalized in the United States annually for pneumococcal pneumonia and pumped full of antibiotics. Still, 40,000 of them die.

This needn't happen. We have had available for more than a decade a safe and effective vaccine against pneumococcal pneumonia, but it is not widely used. During the 1980s, then U.S. Surgeon General C. Everett Koop set a goal of vaccinating 60 percent of the elderly with pneumococcal (and influenza) vaccines. They are recommended for all elderly persons, not just those with chronic medical conditions such as cardiovascular disease, kidney disease or diabetes. Yet we didn't even come close. The last time the Centers for Disease Control surveyed annual immunization rates, in 1985, it was determined that only 10 to 15 percent of the elderly and other high-risk persons had ever received pneumococcal vaccine. In the years since then, says Dr. Fedson, it is unlikely the rate has increased to much more than 20 to 25 percent. The same goal of 60 percent immunized has been repeated for the year 2000, but it too will not be reached without major changes being instituted.

What you can do: First, make certain that if you or any family member is over sixty-five, you receive a pneumococcal vaccine. Second, several studies have shown that if physicians and other health care providers recommend immunization against pneumonia, a high proportion of patients will comply. Ask your doctor if he or she does this as a matter of course. Write the American Medical Association and your local and state medical societies encouraging them to make and enforce an official policy regarding pneumococcal vaccine use.

The other problem is the lack of federal support. Up until now, the government has been reluctant to provide adequate financial support for vaccination programs. Although in 1981 Congress established a Medicare reimbursement program for pneumococcal vaccine, this has not increased its use, probably because the actual level of reimbursement to doctors has been astonishingly low, barely covering the cost of the vaccine. This congressional program, far more sizzle than substance, may actually be providing a financial disincentive for physicians who wish to vaccinate their patients. As genetic engineering is making pneumococcal pneumonia vaccines even more immunologically effective, we can only hope that the Clinton administration will realize how cost-effective it is to prevent pneumonia rather than have to treat it. Contact Hillary Rodham Clinton and your congressional representatives and insist that, as part of any restructuring of our health care system, we need to ensure adequate delivery of this vaccine.

We can, and should, apply these same principles to young children. Pneumococcal pneumonia, while not as common a cause of morbidity or mortality in this age group, still is a significant problem. And it can be greatly avoided by using a similar vaccine, one recently developed and tailored to the subtypes of the pneumococcal bacteria most likely to cause infection in children.

14. SUPPORT RESEARCH INTO NEW VACCINES AND OTHER IMMUNE-ENHANCING SUBSTANCES

When bacteria invade our bodies, in order to attach to a cell, they secrete proteins called adhesins. Vaccines that stimulate production of antibodies against adhesins could be effective in providing immunity to a wide variety of strains of a given bacterial species. A small biotech company called MicroCarb claims to have identified cell receptors and their corresponding adhesins for more than sixty microorganisms and is beginning research on vaccines for several types of bacteria—*Hemophilus influenzae, Streptococcus pneumoniae, Helicobacter pylori* (for ulcers) and *Chlamydia*.

Besides immunological strategies to enhance immune defenses against specific bacteria, there also exists the possibility of bolstering the immune system in a more general way, thereby increasing our resistance to not one bacterial infection, but many or even most. The nonspecific augmenting of immunity is not a new concept. Since the beginning of the century, many studies have demonstrated nonspecific resistance to infection that can be enhanced by the administration of killed microorganisms. Later, it was found that this worked by inducing the production by our immune cells (primarily the T-lymphocytes) of a variety of immune-enhancing proteins called cytokines, such as interferon, interleukin and tumor necrosis factor. The cytokines, in turn, are able to increase the ability of other white blood cells to home in on and kill bacteria. A wide range of serious bacterial infections caused by pneumococcus, *Staphylococcus, Klebsiella* and *Pseudomonas* has been affected by using these cytokines as immunomodulators. This procedure, however, is still in the laboratory. While they have great clinical potential to replace the use of antibiotics in certain situations, the cytokines are still too toxic. More research needs to be done to determine proper doses, to engineer the cytokines better genetically to improve their effectiveness, to evaluate which combinations work best and to see if certain premedications will reduce toxicity without reducing effectiveness.

What you can do: For the antiadhesin vaccines, the biotech industry needs additional investment. If you are in a position to invest, discuss the financial health of MicroCarb with an analyst and also see if there are other companies pursuing the same technology. For the nonspecific modulators, this is an issue that needs additional research support from the National Institutes of Health. Write the director and ask for more dollars to be channeled into immune modulators. Also ask your senators and congressman to help.

15. DEVELOP NEW DRUGS TO FIGHT INFECTIONS AND OVERCOME RESISTANCE

First, all the good news.

In the late 1980s, Dr. Michael Zasloff, professor of pediatrics and chief of molecular biology at the University of Pennsylvania School of Medicine, wondered why African clawed frogs rarely became infected in the dirty water of holding tanks. After some research he discovered the answer in frog skin: a series of proteinlike compounds capable of killing bacteria, protozoa and fungi. He named them magainins.

Only a couple of years later, in 1989, Dr. Zasloff listened to a lecture describing how pregnant dogfish sharks flush their fallopian tubes with seawater to eliminate fetal waste and again wondered how the fetuses were protected from the murky water. Finally, in 1993, he and his graduate student Karen Moore isolated a novel compound from several shark tissues that can kill a wide variety of microorganisms, a steroid compound they dubbed squalamine. He believes the antimicrobial activity of squalamine to be comparable to that of ampicillin.

Dr. Zasloff's ingenuity is but one example of the possibilities that exist for developing anti-infectives that work differently from the standard antibiotics. In fact, his work on magainins has already been expanded by a drug company, Magainin Pharmaceuticals (Dr. Zasloff is executive vice president). The company has been working on a compound called MSI-78, which in 1993 entered FDA trials for the topical treatment of bacterial infections. It is now working to develop a systemic antibacterial compound from squalamine.

Another approach is to find techniques that can eliminate resistance plasmids from bacterial cells—for example, inserting an analogue of an R-factor capable of blocking the expression of resistance to one or more antibiotics. A corollary to this research should be drugs to dislocate the transposons, the even smaller pieces of molecular material that now carry many resistance genes.

We also need more research on the molecular basis of new resistance mechanisms affecting existing antibiotics. The breakthrough in 1992 at Hammersmith Hospital in London on specifically how TB bacteria become resistant to the antibiotic isoniazid is proof that this avenue can yield important results for other antibiotics.

The most exciting area for progress exists in what is called rational drug design, or structure-based drug design. All infectious agents—bacteria, viruses and fungi—encode or carry their own crucial enzymes and DNA, which therefore serve as obvious targets for intervention. In the past decade and a half, the ability to clone and purify these proteins and nucleic acids has improved enormously, to the point where it is now possible to exploit strategies for the discovery and design of a wide variety of inhibitors. According to Dr. Irwin Kuntz, a pharmaceutical chemist at the University of California, San Francisco, structural techniques have also advanced, especially in the area of crystallography and magnetic resonance imaging, which have allowed for the understanding at the three-dimensional level of the bacterial compounds to be inhibited. Taking this information to highly sophisticated computer-aided design programs, scientists can sculpt on screen the exact compound they need.

The first and perhaps most promising opportunity to employ this technique of rational drug design could come as a result of a discovery made early in 1993 at Harvard Medical School that electrified the scientific community. It has been known for some time that it was not possible to determine how bacteria would act in the body by observing and studying how they behave on petri dishes in the laboratory. Too often it would be discovered that an organism that appeared tame in the lab would become a disease-causing terror in animals or humans. It was suspected that such organisms possessed genes—called virulence genes—that somehow remained hidden or inactive until the bacteria were inside the body, at which time the genes would become activated, allowing the microorganisms to cause disease and spread from tissue to tissue.

By using a truly ingenious method of chopping up bacterial DNA into fragments and recombining it in certain sequences, Dr. John Mekalanos and his colleagues were able to uncover the bacterial secrets and identify the virulence genes. This was originally done in a strain of typhoid bacteria that affect only mice, but Dr. Mekalanos feels certain the same techniques can be applied to almost all human bacterial diseases as well.

The first payoff from this research could be the rationally designed development of new drugs to block the virulence genes. This represents such a departure from previous approaches that to call them antibiotics would really be inaccurate; scientists will have to come up with a new name (perhaps antivirulents?). Since the virulence genes—just like all other genes—direct the formation of proteins that carry out their instructions, it will be theoretically possible to develop new vaccines to block the function of the virulence proteins.

Another fruitful result of this discovery, according to Dr. Staffan Normark of Washington University in St. Louis, an expert on the molecular basis of bacterial illness, is the possibility of looking at how the virulence genes behave in different strains of mice. These findings can then be extrapolated to people, to answer the perplexing question of why some organisms cause disease in some people but not in others. To say simply that it is a matter of one having superior resistance to another is too glib. Understanding how our immune systems interact with the virulence genes could provide the answer, leading to yet more innovative ways of resisting bacterial infection without antibiotics.

Now the bad news.

There is not nearly enough support for developing these scientific ideas into drugs that can be used to treat patients. The biotech companies we cited working in the field are too anomalous to make enough of a contribution. We need to get the pharmaceutical industry charged up in a big way. At present, most companies are looking for future profits in areas other than anti-infective compounds. It was estimated in 1992 at a National Institutes of Health workshop that 50 percent of the pharmaceutical industry has either decreased or outright curtailed antimicrobial research. The reason given was that they felt the antibiotic market was glutted. While it may be overcrowded with "me-too" compounds, there are these tremendous new opportunities that need to be encouraged. No doubt, they will be very R&D intensive.

This is where the government comes in. Just as was done for the anticancer drug taxol, there need to be more CRADAs (Cooperative Research and Development Agreements), in which pharmaceutical firms cooperate with government agencies such as the National Institutes of Health. Much of the basic science will be done at the NIH and then brought to market by the private sector, each segment doing what it does best. To provide additional incentives, pharmaceutical companies should be urged to form consortiums and be given additional tax credits and longer patent protection. Even Senator David Pryor of Arkansas, an ardent critic of the pharmaceutical industry, supports this idea, at least in theory. If the pharmaceutical companies don't develop these compounds, who will? Prices can still be controlled by agreement, and in the long run it will save the health care system billions of dollars and millions of lives.

What you can do: The development of new strategies to kill bacteria is a big idea and where much of the future of fighting infection lies. You should strongly encourage your political representatives and Hillary Rodham Clinton to jump on this bandwagon and support CRADAs and the other incentives for the drug industry. Concomitantly, we need a much larger budget at the NIH. Otherwise, all the ingenuity in the world won't transfer to one life saved or one resistant bacterium thwarted.

This, then, with all its ramifications, is the problem facing us today. It is one of enormous magnitude. Bacterial resistance to antibiotics continues to develop inexorably, every day and everywhere in the world, and the number of patients with infections that can't be controlled mounts. Since this process is inherent in the molecular makeup of bacteria, we can't stop it entirely. But by beginning right now to use antibiotics appropriately, we can slow it down. If we do, it will buy us some time to begin intense development and implementation of the alternative methods of thwarting bacteria. If we don't, the consequences are almost too horrible to imagine.

PART TWO:

TOWARD A SOLUTION

I. A Glossary of the Most Commonly Used Antibiotics in Human Therapy

This is a compilation of more than ninety antibiotics grouped according to class, including both the advantages and disadvantages of their therapeutic use. Note that there is often more than one kind of antibiotic that may be effective in treating a given infection. The specific choice depends on a variety of factors, especially the type of bacterium causing the disease. These are discussed in Section II. The drugs are listed by both their generic names and their trade names. Your pharmacist or physician may refer to them either way.

AMINOGLYCOSIDES

Main Use: Some external eye, ear and skin infections; urinary tract infections; septicemia; uncomplicated gonorrhea. Although the aminoglycosides are effective drugs, in recent years resistance has become a serious impediment to therapy. In addition, the use of these drugs is often associated with toxic side effects, especially in the kidney. For this reason, they must be used with caution, if at all, in older people, who frequently have some age-related impairment in kidney function.

GENERIC NAME	TRADE NAME
Amikacin	Amikin
Gentamicin	Garamycin
Kanamycin	Kantrex
Neomycin	Mycifradin, Neobiotic
Netilmicin	Netromycin
Paromomycin	Humatin
Spectinomycin	Trobicin
Streptomycin	No trade name
Tobramycin	Nebcin

ANTITUBERCULOSIS AGENTS

Main Use: Treatment of tuberculosis (and some related organisms that infect patients with suppressed immune systems, especially AIDS patients). The cases of multidrug-resistant TB are usually caused by bacteria resistant to INH, PAS and pyrazinamide, but sometimes rifampin as well.

GENERIC NAME	TRADE NAME
Capreomycin	Capastat
Clofazimine	Lamprene
Cycloserine	Oxamycin, Seromycin
Dapsone	Avlosulfon
Ethambutol	Myambutol
Ethionamide	Trecator
Isoniazid	INH
Para-aminosalicylic acid	PAS
Pyrazinamide	No trade name
Rifabutin	Ansamycin, Mycobutin
Rifampin	Rifadin, Rimactan

CEPHALOSPORINS

Main Use: Cephalosporins have a broad range of antibacterial activity, and are used in prophylaxis or prevention of infection prior to surgical procedures, including cardiovascular and orthopedic procedures and in the treatment of a variety of conditions: pneumonia (both community- and hospital-acquired, mild and severe); meningitis; urinary tract infections; bronchitis; middle ear infections; gonorrhea. They are grouped into categories called generations. In general, with each succeeding generation of cephalosporins, the range of their antibacterial activity broadens. While they are valuable for treating many serious infections, especially hospital-acquired pneumonias, because they have such a wide range of activity the wholesale use of these drugs is more likely to result in the emergence of resistant bacteria.

GENERIC NAME	TRADE NAME
First-Generation Cephalosporins	
Cefadroxil	Duricef
Cefazolin	Ancef, Kefzol
Cefprozil	Cefzil
Cephalexin	Keflex
Cephalothin	Keflin
Cephapirin	Cefadyl
Cephradine	Anspor, Velocef
Second-Generation Cephalosporins	
Cefaclor	Ceclor
Cefamandole	Mandol
Cefmetazole	Zefazone
Cefonicid	Monocid
Ceforanide	Precef
Cefotetan	Cefotan
Cefoxitin	Mefoxin
Cefuroxime	Kefurox, Zinacef

Third-Generation Cephalosporins

Cefixime	Suprax
Cefoperazone	Cefobid
Cefotaxime	Claforan
Cefpiramide	Still investigational drug
Cefpirome	Still investigational drug
Ceftazidime	Fortaz, Ceptaz, others
Ceftizoxime	Cefizox
Ceftriaxone	Rocephin

GLYCOPEPTIDES

Main Use: Endocarditis; pneumonia; meningitis; septicemia; peritonitis; colitis. These antibiotics tend to be toxic and expensive and therefore should be reserved for very serious infections.

GENERIC NAME	TRADE NAME
Teicoplanin	Investigational in U.S.
Vancomycin	Vancocin, Vancor

MACROLIDES

Main Use: Until recently, the only member of this class was erythromycin, which is effective in some forms of pneumonia, both as a primary agent and as an alternative to pencillin in allergic patients. Erythromycin is also used to treat strep throat (again in patients allergic to penicillin), some pelvic infections during pregnancy and some urinary tract infections and as a preventive against infection before colon surgery. Although a safe antibiotic, erythromycin often causes gastrointestinal upset. Recently, two newer relatives have been approved, azithromycin and clarithromycin, which have far fewer effects on the stomach and intestines and which also have a much broader spectrum of activity. They are effective in more types of pneumonia and bronchitis, as well as urinary tract infections, and are being studied as a treatment for Lyme disease. The main advantage of these newer members of the group is that they are able to clear most infections within a much shorter period, usually five days. If these antibiotics are not overused, they could become important not only in the treatment of disease but in the slowing down of emergence of resistant bacteria.

GENERIC NAME	TRADE NAME
Azithromycin	Zithromax
Clarithromycin	Biaxin
Erythromycin	E-mycin, several others

MONOBACTAMS

Main Use: Urinary tract infections (especially complicated ones); lower respiratory tract infections, including pneumonia and bronchitis; septicemia; skin infections, including those associated with postoperative wounds; intra-abdominal infections including peritonitis; and gynecological infections including endometritis. It is available only by injection. Because there is a narrow spectrum of activity, whenever it can be established that the bacteria causing the infection are susceptible to these antibiotics, they are an excellent choice to limit the emergence of antibiotic-resistant bacteria. As the range of bacteria they are effective against tends to overlap that of the aminoglycosides, they are a good alternative in elderly patients and those with impaired kidney function.

GENERIC NAME	TRADE NAME
Aztreonam	Azactam

PENICILLINS

Main Use: Pneumonia; meningitis; gonorrhea (when susceptible); syphilis; strep throat. Since the introduction of penicillin in the 1940s, the different types of this antibiotic have markedly increased. Ninety-five percent of staphylococci bacteria worldwide are resistant to penicillin, and over the past few decades there have become available several penicillin derivatives (such as methicillin) to treat these staph (unless they are also among the growing group resistant to methicillin as well). There are also now many penicillins that have a wide range of antibacterial activity (the prototype was ampicillin), similar to that of the cephalosporins. While this makes the penicillins more useful in general, the chances of antibiotic-resistant strains of bacteria emerging are increased.

GENERIC NAME	TRADE NAME
Penicillin G	Pentids, Pfizerpen
Penicillin V	V-Cillin K
Broad-Spectrum Penicillins	
Amoxicillin	Amoxil, several others
Amoxicillin/clavulanic acid	Augmentin
Amoxicillin/sulbactam	Unasyn
Ampicillin	Polycillin, Omnipen, others
Antipseudomonal Penicillins	
Azlocillin	Azlin
Carbenicillin	Geopen, Pyopen
Mezlocillin	Mezlin
Piperacillin	Pipracil, several others
Ticarcillin	Ticar
Antistaphylococcal Penicillins	
Cloxacillin	Tegopen
Dicloxacillin	Dynapen, Dycill, others
Methicillin	Staphcillin, others
Nafcillin	Unipen, Nafcil
Oxacillin	Prostaphlin, Resistopen, others

QUINOLONES

Main Use: The oldest representative of this group (nalidixic acid) is used exclusively to treat uncomplicated urinary tract infections, such as cystitis (bladder infections). While the newer agents are also effective for simple urinary tract infections, they are also used for more serious complicated urinary infections, such as kidney infections and prostatitis. In addition, they are used for bronchitis, traveler's diarrhea, skin infections, bone infections and sexually transmitted diseases (gonorrhea, chlamydial infection and chancroid). Because of overuse, resistance to ciprofloxacin, notably from methicillin-resistant staph bacteria, has become a serious problem.

GENERIC NAME	TRADE NAME
Ciprofloxacin	Cipro
Enoxacin	Comprecin
Lomefloxacin	Maxaquin
Nalidixic acid	NegGram, Cybis
Norfloxacin	Noroxin
Ofloxacin	Floxin

SULFONAMIDES

Main Use: The sulfas, the first chemotherapeutic agents with significant effectiveness against bacteria without formidable side effects, are still used often today, primarily to treat urinary infections.

GENERIC NAME	TRADE NAME
Sulfacytine	Renoquid
Sulfadiazine	Sulfadiazine
Sulfamethizole	Thiosulfil
Sulfamethoxazole	Gantanol
Sulfasalazine	Azulfidine, Azaline
Sulfisoxazole	Gantrisin, others
Trimethoprim/sulfisoxazole	Bactrim, Septra

TETRACYCLINES

Main Use: Sexually transmitted diseases, especially chlamydial infections; Lyme disease (early stages); some pneumonias; some urinary infections. Resistance to the tetracyclines has been a problem for some time, and resistance to one tetracycline is usually accompanied by resistance to the others.

GENERIC NAME	TRADE NAME
Demeclocycline	Declomycin
Doxycycline	Vibramycin
Methacycline	Rondomycin
Minocycline	Minocin
Oxytetracycline	Terramycin, Urobiotic
Tetracycline	Achromycin

THIENAMYCINS

Main Use: Bone infections; obstetric and gynecological infections; complicated urinary tract infections; intra-abdominal infections; pneumonia; some forms of endocarditis (heart valve infections). These antibiotics, which have only one current representative, are similar to cephalosporins in that they have a broad range of activity against many different bacteria. They are available only by injection and are the most expensive antibiotics on any hospital formulary. For all these reasons, they should be reserved for the treatment of serious conditions.

GENERIC NAME	TRADE NAME
Imipenem	Primaxin

OTHER ANTIBIOTICS

The following list consists of antibiotics that don't fall into a well-defined class. As such, their range of antibacterial activity varies and is given for each individual drug. One of these antibiotics, chloramphenicol, is rarely used anymore, because of the possibility of bone marrow failure.

GENERIC NAME	TRADE NAME	USE
Chloramphenicol	Chloromycetin	typhoid fever
Metronidazole	Flagyl	*Trichomonas* vaginitis; some pneumonia; some meningitis; brain abscess
Nitrofurantoin	Furadantin Macrodantin	urinary infections
Clindamycin	Cleocin	abdominal infections; endocarditis; acne (topical)

II. A Specific Guide to Proper Antibiotic Use

In providing a list of infections and recommended treatments for them, I've tried to balance the need for effective treatment with the need to avoid the emergence of resistant bacteria. The diseases range from the common to the unfamiliar, from relatively mild and uncomplicated to serious and life-threatening. This guide is the safest reference I am aware of for dealing with the need to maintain this balance.

After a brief description of each disease and the most common organisms that could be causing it, there follows a recommended treatment. If the condition is not serious, my advice will almost always be to delay antibiotics until the results of cultures and antibiotic sensitivity tests are available. Knowing what the responsible bacteria are and exactly what antibiotics they are sensitive to takes the guesswork out of treatment and is the best way to avoid the possible emergence of resistant strains.

Unfortunately, diseases don't always come in neat packages. Sometimes, there won't be readily accessible culture material—for example, with an infected gallbladder—or the disease will be severe enough to warrant antibiotic therapy before culture results are available, or both. In those situations, the doctor will have to use his experience as to what the most likely causative organisms are, and what antibiotics are most likely to eradicate the infection. Even here, however, the emphasis in this guide will be on the fewest and narrowest-spectrum antibiotics possible.

For convenience of reference, conditions are listed alphabetically, in most cases according to the part of the body affected. There are a few exceptions, such as Lyme disease, which can involve multiple organs and tissues, and certain other conditions addressed by symptom rather than by location in the body.

INFECTIONS:

BONE

The only infection we need concern ourselves with in bone is osteomyelitis, but there are several varieties and all are serious conditions. Osteomyelitis is almost always caused by bacteria, but occasionally by a fungus or a virus (see the reference to AIDS below). The infection can begin directly in the bone, when bacteria enter through a fracture site or other trauma, or as an extension from another injury, such as a skin ulcer in the foot of a diabetic invading the surrounding bone or a dental infection in the gum extending into the skull. On occasion, especially in children, the infection can be transmitted via the bloodstream from an unknown source into the bone.

The signs and symptoms of osteomyelitis differ according to the specific type, but usually include fever and pain or tenderness over the bone. It can be diagnosed by an elevated white blood count on a blood test and by a bone scan. But to determine the specific cause requires a bacterial culture, from either the blood, bone, or pus from a surrounding abscess. The seriousness of osteomyelitis requires that treatment be instituted immediately, before the culture reports are back, and then adjusted thereafter. In many cases, the initial therapy will have to be in the hospital, with intravenous antibiotics, and then followed by oral antibiotics for several weeks at home. In milder cases, the entire course of treatment can be as an outpatient.

Osteomyelitis in the newborn up to 3 months old

Most common causes   *Staphylococcus aureus*, methicillin-sensitive; *Staphylococcus aureus,* methicillin-resistant; *Streptococcus;* Enterobacteriaceae (a family of gram-negative bacteria).

Best treatment   Must be begun before the results of cultures (taken from the blood) are available. Unfortunately, this calls for the heavy artillery, a sad way for a newborn to begin life. But the consequences of not using these drugs are far worse than using them. Until specific bacteria are identified, the infant should be treated with three antibiotics: vancomycin, a third-generation cephalosporin and rifampin. Once the lab report comes back, one or more antibiotics can be eliminated. (For example, if the bacteria were staph but not methicillin-resistant, the vancomycin and rifampin could be discontinued immediately.)

Osteomyelitis in children from 3 months of age to adult

Most common causes   Staph. aureus, methicillin-resistant; *Staph. aureus*, methicillin-sensitive; *Streptococcus; Hemophilus influenzae.*

Best treatment   Although there is a slight difference in the most likely causes of osteomyelitis in this age group, the treatment plan is the same, again eliminating the vancomycin and the rifampin if the culture report indicates any cause other than methicillin-resistant staph.

Osteomyelitis in an adult IV drug user

The same organisms and treatment regimen as in newborns, except at much higher doses.

Osteomyelitis in an adult (cause not specified)

Most common causes   Staph. aureus, methicillin-resistant; *Staph. aureus*, methicillin-sensitive; *Staph epidermidis; Pseudomonas.*

Best treatment   With the change in the most prevalent organisms causing osteomyelitis in this age group (*Staph. epidermidis* and

Pseudomonas), the antibiotic regimen has to change. Vancomycin still must be used, not only because of the possibility of methicillin-resistant staph, but because of another kind of staph called *Staph. epidermidis*, which is often resistant to methicillin. In those circumstances, the only antibiotic that will touch it is vancomycin. Even this situation is getting worrisome. Because of the necessary increased usage of vancomycin, a few cases of resistance to this antibiotic have surfaced in *Staph. epidermidis*.

Ciprofloxacin, no longer very effective (but sometimes) for methicillin-resistant staph, must be added because of the possibility of *Pseudomonas* as the causative organism. Once again, the physician should adjust the antibiotic regimen as soon as the results of cultures become available. If vancomycin is no longer necessary, either because methicillin-resistant staph is not the cause or because the bacteria are sensitive to ciprofloxacin, the vancomycin should be discontinued immediately. This is wise not only to reduce resistance and preserve vancomycin for life-threatening infections, but also because at the doses necessary in the adult intravenous vancomycin has several toxic side effects (including fever, kidney toxicity and bone marrow suppression) and is prohibitively expensive.

Osteomyelitis in a diabetic with a foot ulcer

Most common causes   Peptostreptococci; anaerobic streptococci; other anaerobic bacteria.

Best treatment   Metronidazole. Also called Flagyl, this antibiotic is quite effective against anaerobic bacteria (those that grow only in the absence of oxygen), and anaerobic bacteria are the most common cause of osteomyelitis in diabetics. Metronidazole generally doesn't cause much of a problem with resistance, but is expensive (fifty dollars a day) and there are often gastrointestinal side effects, including diarrhea, nausea and vomiting and a "furry tongue."

Osteomyelitis in a patient with AIDS

Most common cause   Not caused by bacteria; usually caused by a virus called CMV (cytomegalovirus).

Best treatment   Antiviral drugs, such as ganciclovir or foscarnet.

BRAIN

All infections involving the brain are serious, and many are life-threatening. As such, they should be treated aggressively. Even within that context, however, the possibility of resistance can be given appropriate weight in choosing an antibiotic.

Brain abscess

Brain abscesses can result from opportunistic infections in patients with HIV (see below) or, similar to the way osteomyelitis can arise, by either direct extension from another cranial infection (including osteomyelitis of the skull or face) or from a blood-borne source that lodges in the brain. The tissue dies, fluid is produced and the pressure within the brain increases, causing symptoms resembling a brain tumor. These include headache, nausea, vomiting and seizures. A CT scan or an MRI can usually establish the diagnosis, but for specific cause, fluid from the abscess must be cultured. *As a brain abscess is usually fatal unless treated*, antibiotics must be started immediately, before the culture results are available.

Brain abscess in an HIV-infected patient

MOST COMMON CAUSE   Not caused by bacteria. The most likely cause is toxoplasmosis (*Toxoplasma gondii* is the name of the microorganism, called a protozoan).

BEST TREATMENT   Pyrimethamine. Sometimes sulfadiazine is effective as well; as this drug is cheaper, it should be discussed with the attending physician.

Brain abscess, postoperative

MOST COMMON CAUSES   *Staph. aureus,* methicillin-sensitive and methicillin-resistant; Enterobacteriaceae (gram-negative).

BEST TREATMENT   Begin vancomycin and rifampin, along with a third-generation cephalosporin to cover any gram-negative bacteria as well as methicillin-sensitive staph. Adjust when cultures are available, discontinuing either the cephalosporin (if the cause was a methicillin-resistant staph) or the vancomycin and rifampin (if the cause was anything else).

Brain abscess as an extension of a bone infection in the face or sinuses

MOST COMMON CAUSES   The majority of these abscesses are caused by anaerobic bacteria, such as peptostreptococci and *Bacteroides*, or gram-negative nonanaerobic bacteria called Enterobacteriaceae.

BEST TREATMENT   In order to use only one antibiotic and to cover all possibilities in this life-threatening condition, it is necessary to use imipenem. This is not the type we would like to see used, as it is a very broad-spectrum drug (and also expensive), but the dire circumstances dictate it, at least initially. If the cultures indicate that anaerobic bacteria are the only cause, the imipenem should be discontinued immediately and replaced with metronidazole, which will cover any anaerobic bacteria and lead to far less resistance than imipenem.

Meningitis

Acute meningitis is a genuine medical emergency. With a death rate of about 30 percent (which has changed little in the past twenty-five years), aggressive measures are indicated. Besides initiating antibiotic therapy as soon as meningitis is suspected, the responsible organism should be identified as rapidly as possible. That will allow not only for the appropriate drug to be given if the cause is bacterial but, since sometimes meningitis is caused by viruses, fungi, protozoa or parasites, for the discontinuance of antibiotic therapy altogether.

Meningitis in an adult over sixty years old

MOST COMMON CAUSES   Pneumococcus, gram-negative bacteria (especially *Pseudomonas, E. coli* and Enterobacteriaceae) and *Listeria*.

BEST TREATMENT   The signs of meningitis in the elderly can be subtle. If you are a caregiver and notice fever, irritability, confusion or lassitude, the patient should be taken to the emergency room immediately. The physician will perform a spinal tap, to be sent for culture and a Gram stain, and blood tests. While awaiting the results of these, the doctor should begin intravenous treatment with a third-generation cephalosporin (best choice is probably ceftazidime) and an aminoglycoside, such as gentamicin or tobramycin, to cover all possibilities. Once the lab results are in, the therapy can be changed. If pneumococcus is the cause (highly likely), everything else should be discontinued and a high-dose penicillin given.

Meningitis in an adolescent or adult less than sixty

MOST COMMON CAUSES   Pneumococcus, *Neisseria meningitidis* (meningococcus).

BEST TREATMENT   The signs and symptoms in this age group will usually be better defined and often involve fever, stiff neck, headache and vomiting. Following the spinal tap and blood tests, high doses of intravenous penicillin should begin, to which both pneumococcus and meningococcus are usually sensitive. The results of the tests should confirm the cause and antibiotic sensitivity, so rarely will any change in therapy be indicated.

Meningitis in an infant less than three months old

MOST COMMON CAUSES   E. coli, group B and D streptococci, *Listeria,* herpesvirus type II (many of the organisms which could have inhabited the vagina of the mother).

BEST TREATMENT   As with the elderly, the signs and symptoms of meningitis in newborns are often difficult for either a well-informed parent or even a health professional to discern. If the baby is irritable, has a fever or feeds poorly, it should be suspected, a spinal tap performed, and the condition treated with antibiotics immediately. These should include ampicillin and gentamicin, and when the bacteria sensitivity report is available, be narrowed down to one or the other. If the cause was viral (herpes or another virus), all antibiotics should be stopped immediately.

Meningitis in children three months to ten years

MOST COMMON CAUSES Pneumococcus, meningococcus, *Hemophilus influenzae.*

BEST TREATMENT Although penicillin is the drug of choice for pneumococcus and meningococcus, many cases of meningitis in young children are caused by *Hemophilus*, which is insensitive to penicillin. With increased use of the vaccine against *Hemophilus*, the incidence of cases due to this organism is decreasing, but unless an immediate Gram stain of the spinal fluid is conclusive for another type of bacteria, it is crucial to cover the *Hemophilus* possibility until the culture results are available. Therefore, the best initial therapy is a third-generation cephalosporin, with a switch to penicillin if *Hemophilus* is not the cause.

Meningitis in a patient with AIDS

MOST COMMON CAUSE Usually not a bacterial disease. The cause is almost invariably a fungus called *Cryptococcus*.

BEST TREATMENT Amphotericin B (an antifungal drug).

BREAST

Infection in the breast is relatively rare, and when one develops it often becomes walled off to form an abscess. Abscesses are caused by different organisms, and therefore treated differently, depending on whether they occur immediately after pregnancy or at any other time.

Breast abscess, not associated with pregnancy

MOST COMMON CAUSES *Peptostreptococcus* (anaerobic), several types of *Bacteroides* (also anaerobic), *Staphylococcus aureus* (methicillin-sensitive and -resistant).

BEST TREATMENT Breast abscesses are not life-threatening infections but are serious enough to justify beginning therapy before the specific cause is known. As anaerobic bacteria are the most likely cause of the abscess, treatment should begin with metronidazole. When cultures of the pus-filled breast fluid are available within a couple of days, therapy can be fine-tuned. If the cause is found to be a non-methicillin-resistant staph, the metronidazole should be discontinued and replaced with nafcillin or oxacillin. These penicillin derivatives are also good because they have a relatively narrow spectrum of action and thus don't heavily select for resistant bacteria.

If the cause is found to be methicillin-resistant staph (fortunately, less likely than one that is sensitive), vancomycin will have to be used. But since a breast abscess is not as serious a condition as osteomyelitis, vancomycin shouldn't be started without culture results.

Breast abscess, postpartum

MOST COMMON CAUSES   Staph. aureus, either methicillin-sensitive or methicillin-resistant.

BEST TREATMENT   Initiate with nafcillin or oxacillin. If cultures indicate a methicillin-resistant staph, a shift to vancomycin will be necessary.

EAR

Infections in the ear can involve either the external ear canal (otitis externa) or the middle ear (otitis media) and can range in severity from very mild external infections, necessitating only topical treatment, to severe middle ear infections which may require hospitalization.

External otitis ("swimmer's ear")

MOST COMMON CAUSES   All are gram-negative bacteria: Proteus, Pseudomonas and Enterobacteriaceae.

BEST TREATMENT   Whether the genesis of external otitis is swimming or not, virtually all of these infections are caused by the same bacteria and always treated with topical ear drops, usually Cortisporin.

Since there is little absorption of these antibiotics into the body, and hence little selection for resistant strains, cultures are not necessary here.

External otitis in a diabetic

MOST COMMON CAUSES   *Pseudomonas aeruginosa.*

BEST TREATMENT   This is the only exception to the topical treatment of external ear infections. In diabetics, this can be a severe condition (it is sometimes even called malignant otitis externa). As such, it needs to be treated with systemic antibiotics, gentamicin being the best choice.

Otitis media, acute

MOST COMMON CAUSES   *Streptococcus pneumoniae* (pneumococcus), *Hemophilus influenzae, Branhamella catarrhalis.*

BEST TREATMENT   Once middle ear infection is diagnosed by an ear exam with an otoscope (looking especially for fluid against the eardrum), antibiotic therapy should be begun promptly. Because removing fluid from the middle ear is a difficult chore for the physician and painful for the patient, cultures are rarely taken. Most responsible bacteria are still sensitive to amoxicillin or ampicillin, and these are the initial treatments of choice. However, the number of resistant strains is increasing, and if the infection doesn't clear up within three days (fever and pain disappear), it may be assumed that the bacteria are resistant (probably *H. influenzae* or *Branhamella*) and the drug should be promptly switched to amoxicillin-clavulanate or a third-generation cephalosporin. If the resistant bacteria are picked up this quickly, most experts believe there is at present no danger of extension to meningitis. Therapy should then be continued for ten days.

Otitis media, chronic or recurrent

MOST COMMON CAUSES   Pneumococcus, *Hemophilus, Branhamella.*

BEST TREATMENT   Although the causative organisms are almost the same as with acute otitis media, the treatment is different. There is

debate in the scientific literature as to whether prophylactic antibiotics (amoxicillin or sulfisoxazole) in winter and early spring are
valuable, the most recent studies indicating that there is little merit
in this approach. For children over two years, vaccinating against
pneumococcus may be helpful. If nothing else works, the surgical
placing of tubes resembling small collar buttons in the eardrum may
prevent the fluid buildup. This is clearly a condition with many treatment options and should be thoroughly discussed with one's physician before the wholesale use of antibiotics.

EYE

The most common eye disease in the Western Hemisphere is conjunctivitis, an infection of the membrane lining the eye, and something most of us experience at least once. Other infections involve
the eyelid (blepharitis and styes), the cornea (keratitis) and the interior of the eye cavity (endophthalmitis).

Conjunctivitis

MOST COMMON CAUSES   The most common sign of conjunctivitis is
redness of the conjunctiva, hence the popular designation "pink
eye." The majority of cases of conjunctivitis are due to viruses, but
bacteria are a close second and should be suspected whenever there
is a pus discharge from the eye, which should be cultured. The usual
culprits are pneumococcus and *Staphylococcus* in adults and these
organisms plus *Hemophilus influenzae* in children.

BEST TREATMENT   Most times bacterial conjunctivitis is mild and
self-limiting and therefore requires only topical drugs such as neomycin or sulfa. The one exception is conjunctivitis secondary to gonorrhea, due either to self-inoculation from a genital infection or, in
the special case of newborns, to an infection transmitted from the
vaginal canal during birth. Cultures will be diagnostic, but if the
doctor suspects gonorrhea from the history, an injection of a third-
generation cephalosporin (for an adult) or instillation of a tetracycline ointment (newborn) is important.

Blepharitis

MOST COMMON CAUSES   Although it can be uncomfortable and unsightly to have one's eyelids and eyelashes itchy, crusty and stuck together, blepharitis is not a serious infection. In some cases, mascara use has been implicated as an initiating factor. The bacteria involved are almost always staphylococci.

BEST TREATMENT   Erythromycin or bacitracin ointment.

Stye

MOST COMMON CAUSE   Known medically as a hordeolum, a stye is an infection of the eyelid caused almost always by staphylococci.

BEST TREATMENT   Since the infection is so localized, hot soaks are usually sufficient. Sometimes erythromycin ointment is needed.

Keratitis

MOST COMMON CAUSES   Many causes of corneal inflammation are noninfectious, for example, trauma (often from contact lenses) and allergic reactions. When infectious, bacteria are the causes about three-quarters of the time, although viruses, fungi and parasites can be responsible as well. Corneal infections are potentially sight-threatening and need to be regarded seriously and treated promptly. The most commonly involved bacteria are staph or *Pseudomonas*, and loss of sight can occur within twenty-four hours after an untreated infection by either of them.

BEST TREATMENT   Because of the severity of the condition, the patient will often need to be hospitalized, especially if there is significant ulceration of the cornea. If the physician feels the chances for perforation are great, antibiotics by injection should be started, usually a third-generation cephalosporin. In other instances, the antibiotics can be given topically as a solution or administered under the conjunctiva, a painful procedure but one that delivers a higher concentration of the drug. A third-generation cephalosporin can be used here as well.

Endophthalmitis

MOST COMMON CAUSES   This condition is often a complication of eye surgery, including cataract removal, surgical procedures for glaucoma, and corneal transplantation. Even here, however, the incidence is low, less than one percent of cases. When it does occur, it develops suddenly and progresses rapidly, involving swelling, redness and cloudiness of the entire eye. The bacteria usually responsible are staphylococci, frequently resistant to methicillin. If enough of a discharge is present, a bacterial culture can be taken, but whether this is done or not, antibiotic treatment should begin immediately.

BEST TREATMENT   Until proven to be a non-methicillin-resistant staph, vancomycin should be instilled directly into the chamber of the eye known as the vitreous. If culture results indicate a methicillin-sensitive staph, the antibiotic should be changed to a cephalosporin.

FEVER

Although fever is frequently a sign of infection, it is not always a sign of a bacterial infection. In fact, most fevers will be viral. Unless there is strong reason to suspect a bacterial origin of the fever (such as signs of meningitis or pneumonia), the appropriate course to follow is a thorough diagnostic work-up. With the rare exception of a patient whose white blood count is extremely low (such as an AIDS or cancer patient), antibiotics should not be administered without knowing the cause.

FOOT

Cellulitis

MOST COMMON CAUSES   Cellulitis is an acute spreading infection of the skin that often extends deep enough to involve the subcutaneous tissues. In most cases, streptococci or *Staphylococcus aureus* is the cause, but in diabetics anaerobic bacteria can be responsible or, after a nail puncture, *Pseudomonas*.

BEST TREATMENT Begin with Flagyl (for anaerobic bacteria) along with a third-generation cephalosporin or ciprofloxacin. Take a culture if possible and alter according to results. If only staph, shift to methicillin; if only strep, shift to penicillin; if only anaerobic bacteria, treat with Flagyl; if *Pseudomonas*, treat only with a third-generation cephalosporin.

GALLBLADDER

Although cholecystitis—inflammation of the gallbladder, usually secondary to or associated with gallstones—remains an extremely common condition, bacterial infection is rare. When it occurs, not only is the gallbladder seeded with bacteria, but often the bile ducts as well. The appropriate material to culture to identify specific bacteria is bile, but since bile is not readily accessible, cultures are rarely taken unless at the time of surgery. If the patient shows signs of infection, such as fever, it is justified for the physician to begin empiric antibiotic treatment. As in all cases of appropriate empiric therapy, the choice of antibiotics should be based on what previous studies have shown to be the most likely bacteria causing the infection. If the patient appears severely ill, the infection may have extended beyond the gallbladder and bile ducts into the bloodstream, a condition known as sepsis. In that case, blood cultures can be taken to try to identify the causative bacteria, but it is imperative to institute antibiotics immediately.

MOST COMMON CAUSES There are a variety of bacteria that can cause gallbladder infection, with or without sepsis. Most of them are anaerobic types, including species of *Clostridium* (members of this genus can also cause tetanus and botulism) and *Bacteroides*. Besides anaerobic bacteria, a member of the streptococcus group called enterococcus may be responsible. These organisms are becoming increasingly important in both community and hospital-acquired abdominal infections and must be taken into consideration when deciding on the appropriate antibiotics.

BEST TREATMENT   Imipenem and either ampicillin/sulbactam or ampicillin/clavulanic acid will cover all possibilities. If a blood culture is taken, the therapy may be able to be narrowed when the results are available, perhaps eliminating the very broad spectrum imipenem. If not, all drugs should be continued until the patient improves.

GASTROINTESTINAL TRACT

Infections of the gastrointestinal tract can occur anywhere from the mouth to the anus. The mouth is covered under its own heading; the remainder of the conditions listed here involve the stomach and the small and large intestines.

Duodenal ulcer

MOST COMMON CAUSES   Duodenal ulcer is also sometimes called peptic ulcer. In the past few years, the thinking about ulcers in the medical community has undergone a remarkable transformation. It is now believed that the most common cause of duodenal ulcers is bacteria called *Helicobacter pylori*. Excess stomach acid production and a reduced resistance to this acid by the lining of the intestine, previously thought to be the predominant factors, are still regarded as important, but they now take somewhat of a back seat to *Helicobacter*. Naturally this will affect treatment. Physicians now have at their disposal a number of new noninvasive tests to detect the presence of *Helicobacter,* including an inexpensive blood test. If the bacteria are identified and ulcer symptoms are present, the current thinking is to try to eradicate the *Helicobacter*.

BEST TREATMENT   The antibiotic that has been studied most, and therefore the one recommended, is amoxicillin. In addition, appropriate acid-inhibiting drugs should be used. The usual choice will be ranitidine (Zantac) or cimetidine (Tagamet), but a more powerful and specific acid inhibitor, omeprazole (Prilosec), may be even better, as it seems to have antibacterial properties of its own.

Dysentery

Dysentery, an acute infection of the large intestine, can range in severity from mild, requiring little or no therapy, to life-threatening. The nature of the dysentery is often determined by underlying conditions.

Mild dysentery

MOST COMMON CAUSES   If the only symptom is diarrhea without obvious blood, with no fever or white blood cells present when the doctor performs, or has the lab perform, a microscopic examination of the stool, the dysentery is probably caused by a virus. Stool cultures should be sent to the lab anyway, because the other possible cause is the common intestinal bacterium *E. coli*.

BEST TREATMENT   Initially, it should be assumed that this is a viral infection and no antibiotics are necessary. Here is a situation where you should question your doctor if antibiotics are recommended. If the cause is *E. coli*, the lab will report it within a few days and antibiotics can be started then if necessary. The lab will also report the results of sensitivity tests, so no guesswork will be needed by the doctor. Most strains will be sensitive to ampicillin.

Severe dysentery

MOST COMMON CAUSES   Severe dysentery is more common among travelers to developing countries, where the bacteria are usually disseminated by a contaminated water supply. In contrast to mild viral or *E. coli* dysentery, someone with severe dysentery will usually have a fever and explosive bloody stools which contain many white blood cells on microscopic exam, indicative of a bacterial infection. Since a great deal of fluid and electrolytes may be lost via the diarrhea, hospitalization is often required. Stool cultures will demonstrate the bacterial cause within a few days, but this can be a life-threatening situation and antibiotics must be started immediately, administered intravenously along with the fluid replacement. The most likely causes are *Shigella, Vibrio cholerae* (in this case, the dysentery is cholera) and bacteria called *Campylobacter jejuni*.

BEST TREATMENT   Sensitivity reports will be available with the results of the stool cultures. In the meantime, it is best to begin with ciprofloxacin. If the organisms show susceptibility to doxycycline, the antibiotic should then be switched to this older and much cheaper drug. There will, however, be many resistant strains, especially of *Shigella*, the bacterium in which multiple antibiotic resistance was first discovered in the 1950s.

Dysentery in a patient with AIDS

MOST COMMON CAUSES   As with most other infections in AIDS patients, the cause is opportunistic viruses, fungi or parasites, not common bacterial pathogens. In this case cytomegalovirus, parasites called *Giardia* or *Entamoeba,* or a fungus called *Cryptosporidium* is the most likely culprit.

BEST TREATMENT   No antibiotics called for. Antiviral, antifungal and antiparasitic drugs should be used.

Dysentery in an infant

MOST COMMON CAUSES   Depending on the age of the infant, the dysentery might have been contracted while in the hospital or else from the environment. In either case, the most likely cause is *E. coli*. But in contrast to mild dysentery in an adult, an *E. coli*–induced dysentery in an infant can be a serious condition. More fluid can be lost from a system whose balance is more delicate.

BEST TREATMENT   Until stool cultures are available, a third-generation cephalosporin, ceftriaxone, is the drug to which most strains of *E. coli* will be sensitive. Naturally it is to be given intravenously.

Traveler's diarrhea

MOST COMMON CAUSES   Many of the same bacteria that cause the severe form of dysentery can cause traveler's diarrhea, but this is not as serious a condition. Fluid loss is generally much less, and there is often no blood in the stool. The organisms most frequently involved are *Shigella, Campylobacter,* some species of *Salmonella* and sometimes *E. coli*.

BEST TREATMENT   If one is traveling, stool cultures may not be feasible, and treatment will have to be empiric. The best antibiotic under those circumstances is either ciprofloxacin or floxacin, but in a foreign country these will be difficult, if not impossible, to find. The combination sulfa drug sulfamethoxazole/trimethoprim is a reasonable second choice, although more and more bacteria from foreign countries, especially Mexico, are turning up resistant to this antibiotic. If sulfa/trimethoprim is started and symptoms don't subside within a couple of days, it will be too late to do a stool culture. Even when antibiotics don't cure, they can suppress the bacteria enough to invalidate subsequent cultures. If this happens, as soon as one has access to a physician in a more developed country, the antibiotic regimen should be changed to ciprofloxacin or floxacin.

Typhoid fever

MOST COMMON CAUSES   Fortunately, the chances of encountering this highly dangerous and still sometimes fatal disease are small. Typhoid is usually spread either by the water supply or by asymptomatic carriers (like "Typhoid Mary" from earlier in this century). It is almost never seen in the developed world anymore, and anyone traveling to an endemic area is required to be immunized against typhoid fever. When it does occur, the bacterial cause is *Salmonella typhi*. The best way to diagnose typhoid is in the early stages, from a stool culture.

BEST TREATMENT   The treatment of typhoid fever is one of the few circumstances left where the use of the potentially toxic antibiotic chloramphenicol is justified. If one is unlucky enough to be stricken in a Third World country, the physicians there should have a much higher index of suspicion than in a developed country, so the chances of getting the appropriate treatment are probably better than one might think, even if a stool culture isn't performed.

Ulcerative colitis

MOST COMMON CAUSES   Although specific bacteria have never been identified as a cause of ulcerative colitis (the actual cause remains unknown), for reasons not well understood many patients do respond to treatment with an antibacterial agent.

BEST TREATMENT   Along with other drugs, the sulfa drug sulfasalazine is frequently used.

GENITAL TRACT

While most bacterial infections of the genital tract are specific to either males or females, there are a few that are "unisex."

Anogenital warts

MOST COMMON CAUSE   Also sometimes called venereal warts because they are usually contracted through sexual contact, these are not bacterial infections at all, but are a viral condition, caused by the human papillomavirus.

BEST TREATMENT   No antibiotics are indicated. Topical treatment with a solution called podophyllin resin or 5-fluorouracil. Anogenital warts should not be left untreated, especially in women, as some strains of papillomavirus have been implicated in cancer of the cervix.

Vaginitis

MOST COMMON CAUSES   The common symptom of bacterial vaginitis is a malodorous vaginal discharge, usually yellow-tinged. The most likely bacteria present will be anaerobic and include *Peptostreptococcus* and *Bacteroides*. By doing a Gram stain of the discharge, a physician can get an idea of the cause, as peptostreptococci are gram-positive and *Bacteroides* are gram-negative. Treatment can be started but a culture should also be done to confirm what the Gram stain showed and to determine antibiotic sensitivity.

BEST TREATMENT   If the patient is not pregnant, metronidazole (Flagyl) should be started. In a pregnant woman, clindamycin is a better choice. The antibiotics can be adjusted when the culture results are available.

Trichomonal vaginitis

MOST COMMON CAUSE   This is a specific (and common) type of vaginitis, caused by the organisms called *Trichomonas vaginalis*, which really aren't bacteria but protozoa. The characteristic symptom of trichomoniasis is a copious foamy vaginal discharge.

BEST TREATMENT   If the patient describes the typical discharge and/or the doctor is able to identify the organism on a slide, treatment should begin with metronidazole (Flagyl). This antibiotic should not, however, be used in pregnant women, who should be treated instead with a saline douche.

Candidal vaginitis

MOST COMMON CAUSE   Another very common vaginal infection also not caused by bacteria. The offender here is the yeast *Candida*. The tipoff is vaginal itching and a thick, cheesy discharge.

BEST TREATMENT   Antibiotics, either topical or systemic, are not indicated. Antifungal drugs such as nystatin are the appropriate treatment.

Cervicitis

MOST COMMON CAUSES   Whereas vaginitis is often not a sexually transmitted infection (unless it is part of a cervical infection), bacterial infections of the cervix frequently are. The most common causes are gonorrhea (the responsible bacteria are *Neisseria gonorrhoeae*), or *Chlamydia*. The prominent sign is a discharge similar to that seen with vaginitis, and often the patient can't tell where the discharge is coming from. An exam by a doctor, including a Gram stain, may lead to identification, but these bacteria are often difficult to find, especially in women. Whether or not bacteria are found on a Gram stain, a culture of the material should be done.

BEST TREATMENT   Since an infection of the cervix has the potential to spread upward into the fallopian tubes and the uterus, it should be regarded seriously and treatment begun immediately. If the offending organism can't be positively identified on a Gram stain of the discharge, the best antibiotic to use is the quinolone ofloxacin.

This is an expensive drug and one to which resistance is mounting much faster than we would like, but conditions warrant its use, as it is the drug that best covers both bacterial possibilities. When the culture results are available, a more specific drug can be used to treat either gonorrhea or *Chlamydia*. For gonorrhea, the sensitivity will probably indicate that a third-generation cephalosporin is best. It has been almost twenty years since gonococci were exquisitely sensitive to penicillin, and many are now resistant to tetracycline as well. If the cause is *Chlamydia,* the chances of the bacteria being tetracycline-sensitive are greater and the regimen can be switched to doxycycline. If the lab report indicates doxycycline-resistant *Chlamydia,* a new erythromycinlike antibiotic called azithromycin is the best choice.

Chancroid

MOST COMMON CAUSE   Chancroid is a relatively uncommon sexually transmitted disease that causes an ulceration of either the male or female genitalia. The ulceration somewhat resembles the characteristic lesion or chancre of syphilis, hence the name chancroid. The only bacterial cause of chancroid is an organism called *Hemophilus ducreyi,* which can be identified either by a culture of the ulceration or by the clinical suspicion of a good doctor.

BEST TREATMENT   Before culture and sensitivity results are available, erythromycin is the best choice. If the bacteria turn up resistant to erythromycin, one of its newer and more expensive relatives, azithromycin or clarithromycin, will probably work. Another antibiotic to which these bacteria will probably be sensitive is ciprofloxacin.

Early syphilis

MOST COMMON CAUSE   The only cause of syphilis is the spirochete *Treponema pallidum* (called a spirochete because of its corkscrew-like appearance under the microscope; another spirochete is the bacterium that causes Lyme disease). Like gonorrhea and other sexually transmitted diseases, the incidence of syphilis has been rising in recent years. If syphilis can be diagnosed in an early stage (for example, by the characteristic chancre on either the male or female genitalia), antibiotic treatment is invariably effective. It is when syphilis goes untreated and enters the later stages that it becomes a much more serious and sometimes fatal disease.

BEST TREATMENT   Early syphilis is one of the few bacterial diseases that can still be treated with older, cheaper antibiotics. *Treponema pallidum* remains completely sensitive to penicillin, which can be administered in one intramuscular injection or by mouth for ten days. If the patient is allergic to penicillin, erythromycin or doxycycline taken for ten days is a good second choice.

Syphilis of more than one year's duration

MOST COMMON CAUSE   *Treponema pallidum.*

BEST TREATMENT   The only difference in the treatment regimen from early syphilis is the length and strength. Instead of just one injection of penicillin, three, given at weekly intervals, are called for. If doxycycline is to be used, four weeks of therapy are needed to eradicate the bacteria.

Neurosyphilis

MOST COMMON CAUSE   *Treponema pallidum.*

BEST TREATMENT   Injectable penicillin, several doses over several weeks. If the patient is allergic to penicillin, chloramphenicol, a more powerful drug, rather than doxycycline is the antibiotic of choice.

Syphilis in a patient with HIV

MOST COMMON CAUSE   *Treponema pallidum.*

BEST TREATMENT   Same as for a patient without HIV, except many experts recommend using a higher dose of penicillin.

Congenital syphilis

MOST COMMON CAUSE   *Treponema pallidum,* acquired by an infant as the result of the mother being infected.

BEST TREATMENT   Intravenous penicillin every eight hours for ten days, without missing a single day. If this regimen is followed, the infant should have no residual effects of the syphilis.

Urethritis

MOST COMMON CAUSES   The main symptom of urethritis (an inflammation of the urethra, the canal that carries urine from the bladder) is burning on urination. The most commonly involved bacteria are gonococci or *Chlamydia*. The difference between the two is usually easier to discern in men because in male gonorrhea the burning is often accompanied by a pus-containing discharge that can be examined under the microscope and then cultured. Unless there is also an infection of the cervix, gonorrhea frequently causes no discharge in women. Culture will be necessary to home in on the specific cause.

BEST TREATMENT   This is a condition that should be treated before culture results are available, as the complications can be serious, especially of gonorrhea. If gonococci can be identified from a Gram stain, a third-generation cephalosporin should be the antibiotic used. If the bacteria can't be identified at the time of examination, then azithromycin, which can kill both gonococci and *Chlamydia,* is the best drug. But this is a new drug, and in order to reduce the possibility of future resistance, azithromycin should be used only under these specific circumstances. If a culture identifies *Chlamydia* sensitive to doxycycline, the antibiotic should be changed immediately.

Prostatitis

MOST COMMON CAUSES   As with urethritis, the most common causes are gonococci and *Chlamydia*. A discharge may or not be present.

BEST TREATMENT   Without specific identification, azithromycin should be used, then changed to either a cephalosporin (for gonorrhea) or doxycycline (for *Chlamydia*) when culture reports are available.

Endometritis

MOST COMMON CAUSES   This is an infection of the lining of the uterus that usually occurs postpartum. If it occurs within forty-eight hours of a cesarean section, *Chlamydia* is the likely cause, with several anaerobic bacteria close seconds. If the infection occurs several weeks later, the cause is almost always *Chlamydia*.

BEST TREATMENT   Later-occurring endometritis is rarely serious. Besides discontinuing nursing, doxycycline treatment will usually cure the condition. Endometritis immediately postpartum, on the other hand, can be a serious condition. If a discharge is present, it should be stained on the spot and then cultured. Treatment, however, should be instituted immediately and may have to remain empirical if no material is available for culture. The antibiotics to begin with are imipenem to cover any anaerobic bacteria and azithromycin for the *Chlamydia*. If cultures are performed and specific bacteria are identified, one of the two antibiotics can be discontinued, or perhaps the azithromycin changed to doxycycline.

Epididymoorchitis

MOST COMMON CAUSES   This tongue-twister is the name for infection of the epididymis (the organ that stores sperm) and the testes (the organs that produce sperm). As with several other infections of the male and female genital tracts, the most common causes are *Neisseria gonorrhoeae* and *Chlamydia*,

BEST TREATMENT   It may not be possible to obtain material for culture, so treatment will have to be empirical. First the possible gonorrhea (the more serious of the two conditions) should be treated with a third-generation cephalosporin, followed by doxycycline (for *Chlamydia*) if there is no improvement. If there is still no improvement, a doxycycline-resistant *Chlamydia* can be assumed and azithromycin tried.

HAND

Paronychia

MOST COMMON CAUSES   Paronychia is an infection of the nail and the nail bed. It is frequently caused by nail biting or a manicure. The bacteria involved are usually staphylococci, most of which are methicillin-sensitive.

BEST TREATMENT   Methicillin or one of the other antistaphylococcal penicillins.

HEART

Most infections of the heart involve the valves and are called endocarditis. We also address one infection of the pericardium, the sac that covers the heart.

Infective endocarditis

MOST COMMON CAUSES   Common presenting symptoms are fever and a heart murmur. The bacteria are identified by a series of blood cultures, from samples drawn at specific intervals. The most common causes are several types of streptococci, including enterococci.

BEST TREATMENT   This is a serious, potentially life-threatening disease and therefore treatment must be instituted before the results of the blood cultures are available. Most of the strep will be sensitive to penicillin, but enterococci and staph often aren't. Treatment should begin with either ampicillin/sulbactam or ampicillin/clavulanic acid, which kill both strep and enterococci. If cultures reveal that penicillin-sensitive streptococci are the cause, the antibiotic should immediately be switched.

Infective endocarditis in a prosthetic heart valve

MOST COMMON CAUSES   Different bacteria colonize artificial heart valves, usually methicillin-sensitive or methicillin-resistant staphylococci, as well as bacteria called *Staph. epidermidis*. These bacteria have a special affinity for catheters, valves and other synthetic material. In addition, *Candida* are being identified more and more as causes of this type of endocarditis.

BEST TREATMENT   This is a time when heavy antibiotics are necessary. Until blood cultures are available, the possibility that the infection is caused by methicillin-resistant staph or *Staph. epidermidis* must be accounted for. The only antibiotic that can be used is vancomycin, usually in combination with rifampin. In addition, the antifungal drug amphotericin should be given to cover a possible *Candida* cause. Therapy can be fine-tuned when culture reports are ready. If, for example, the cause is found to be methicillin-sensitive staph, all the other drugs should be discontinued in favor of methicillin or a related antibiotic.

Infective endocarditis in an IV drug user

MOST COMMON CAUSES   The possibilities here run the gamut from both kinds of staph to all types of strep and *Pseudomonas*. Many of these bacteria are extremely difficult to eradicate, and treatment is made more difficult by the debilitated state of the drug user.

BEST TREATMENT   Once again, the heavy artillery must be used until the specific bacteria are identified. Vancomycin, gentamicin and trimethoprim/sulfa will cover all possibilities, and treatment can be adjusted when culture reports are available.

Acute pericarditis

MOST COMMON CAUSES   Acute pericarditis can occur following a heart attack or for an unknown reason. Often the cause is viral, but when bacteria are involved, the culprits are usually staphylococci (methicillin-sensitive and -resistant), streptococci or Enterobacteriaceae. Chest pain, shortness of breath and fever are the common symptoms, and a characteristic sound heard with the stethoscope, a pericardial "friction rub," is the tip-off.

BEST TREATMENT   Pericarditis following a heart attack is almost never caused by bacteria, and antibiotics are not warranted. In other cases, blood cultures may be helpful, but treatment should be started empirically and may have to be continued that way if no culture material is positive. Because of the serious nature of the disease and the types of bacteria involved, the antibiotics vancomycin, rifampin and a third-generation cephalosporin will have to be used.

KIDNEY

The most common urinary tract infection isn't really a kidney infection at all, but a bladder infection (called cystitis). But since untreated bladder infections can progress to kidney infections, it's appropriate to discuss them in the same category.

Uncomplicated cystitis

MOST COMMON CAUSES   At least one in five women will have a urinary tract infection during her life. Approximately 80 percent of simple bladder infections are caused by *E. coli,* but in recent years the percentage due to other gram-negative Enterobacteriaceae and enterococci (members of the streptococcus family) has been increasing. By doing a Gram stain and a dipstick of the urine, looking for the presence of a white blood cell enzyme indicative of bacterial infection, a physician can get a pretty good idea of what the cause of the bladder infection is. Culture and sensitivity tests will be definitive.

BEST TREATMENT   If there is dipstick evidence of a bacterial infection, the best antibiotic to start with is ampicillin or amoxicillin. All bacteria except Enterobacteriaceae that aren't *E. coli* should be quite sensitive to either drug. If the culture turns out to grow Enterobacteriaceae, then the antibiotic can be switched to either gentamicin or a third-generation cephalosporin, or even ciprofloxacin. The current practice of many doctors prescribing these drugs right off the bat both is expensive and invites resistance.

Recurrent cystitis

MOST COMMON CAUSES   Recurrent cystitis is defined as three or more episodes of uncomplicated urinary tract infections in a year. Although it is not well understood why some women have recurrent urinary infections, the hormonal changes of menopause and the sagging of the bladder in older women are two predisposing factors.

The bacteria responsible are generally the same as for nonrecurrent cystitis.

Best treatment There is a growing move among some physicians to give women who have demonstrated recurrent cystitis a supply of antibiotics so they can self-treat at the first sign. The rationale behind this is that they can get a head start on preventing extension of the infection into the kidney. While this may, in fact, work for selected patients, as a general policy it is likely to promote resistant bacteria. Most women are given Pyridium, a drug that relieves burning, along with their antibiotics. Hence, they usually feel better within a day. Even though the antibiotics may have to be taken for only five days, the temptation for many would be to discontinue their drug too early, a subtherapeutic course. Unless the doctor feels confident the patient will take the entire dose, it is better for the treatment to be more closely monitored.

Acute pyelonephritis

Most common causes In contrast to cystitis, pyelonephritis (kidney infection) often causes fever, chills and pain or tenderness in the flank overlying the kidney. It is potentially a serious infection. *E. coli* and other Enterobacteriaceae are the most common causes.

Best treatment The patient will frequently need to be hospitalized. Here it is not advisable to wait for the culture report before making certain that all bacteria are covered. The best antibiotic for this is ceftriaxone, a third-generation cephalosporin given by injection only. When the causative bacteria have been identified, the drug can perhaps be shifted to more narrow-spectrum therapy, such as gentamicin or aztreonam. The blood levels of ampicillin or amoxicillin achievable are not great enough to warrant using them for a condition this serious.

LYME DISEASE

Most common causes The only causative organism of Lyme disease is the spirochete *Borrelia burgdorferi,* transmitted to humans by the bite of a deer tick. Although research should soon provide the means for identifying B. *burgdorferi* in tissues and body fluids, this is not yet available. Doctors presently must rely on a blood test that measures antibodies to the organism, which is helpful but indirect. The other sign is the presence of the characteristic bull's-eye rash at the site of a tick bite, which occurs in about three of four cases. If either or both of these conditions exist, treatment should begin.

BEST TREATMENT   Treatment of Lyme disease in the early stages is generally highly successful. Tetracycline, doxycycline and amoxicillin are equally effective. There are also studies being conducted as to whether either or both of the new erythromycinlike drugs, azithromycin or clarithromycin, work as well. The advantage of these antibiotics is that the required course of treatment is much shorter, usually only five days as compared with two to three weeks for the other antibiotics. Because the Lyme spirochete has shown little resistance to any of these antibiotics, some physicians believe that simply living in an endemic area (primarily the Northeast) and being bitten by a deer tick is justification for treatment, but this hardly seems prudent. Rather than push our luck, only suspected cases should get antibiotics. Don't accept antibiotics from your doctor unless you have the rash or a positive blood test.

Lyme disease with arthritis

MOST COMMON CAUSE   *Borrelia burgdorferi.*

BEST TREATMENT   Once Lyme disease has progressed to the point where specific organ systems are involved, treatment must be for longer periods, sometimes with different antibiotics and sometimes by injection. Even here, most patients will still be completely cured. If doxycycline or amoxicillin is taken by mouth, the regimen is now for thirty days. If the patient is very sick, or if medication by mouth has been ineffective, injections of either penicillin or ceftriaxone are the treatment of choice. Ask for penicillin, as it is more narrow spectrum.

Cardiac Lyme disease

MOST COMMON CAUSE   *Borrelia burgdorferi.*

BEST TREATMENT   In about 10 percent of patients with untreated Lyme disease, heart abnormalities develop. They range from relatively mild, such as a nonthreatening rhythm disturbance, to a more serious inflammation of the heart muscle and heart enlargement. Mild cases can be handled with oral doxycycline or amoxicillin; more severe involvement requires injectable penicillin or ceftriaxone.

Neurologic Lyme disease

MOST COMMON CAUSE   *Borrelia burgdorferi.*

BEST TREATMENT   Bell's palsy, an inflammation of the facial nerve which usually is one-sided and causes drooping of the mouth, is the most common neurological manifestation of Lyme disease and is almost always cured with doxycycline or amoxicillin by mouth for thirty days. If neurological involvement is more severe, such as a meningitis, intravenous penicillin or ceftriaxone is needed.

MOUTH

Cellulitis in children less than five years old

MOST COMMON CAUSES   Cellulitis in the mouth of a young child is a serious condition, often following on the heels of a tame upper respiratory infection, and treatment should begin immediately. Although blood cultures and cultures from the infection site should be taken for confirmation, in almost all cases the causative organism is *Hemophilus influenzae.*

BEST TREATMENT   The child needs to be hospitalized and treated intravenously with the third-generation cephalosporin ceftriaxone. Almost all strains of *H. influenzae* are still sensitive, a perfect example of why these broad-spectrum antibiotics should not be used frivolously, but retained for conditions such as these.

Infection following dental work

MOST COMMON CAUSES   These infections are invariably due to anaerobic bacteria, including peptostreptococci and *Fusobacterium.*

BEST TREATMENT   All are sensitive to penicillin.

Infection following dental work in an immunocompromised patient

MOST COMMON CAUSES   In compromised patients, such as those with AIDS, the infection is almost always due to a fungus, *Candida*.

BEST TREATMENT   No antibiotics indicated. Treat with antifungal drugs amphotericin B, fluconazole or ketoconazole.

RESPIRATORY TRACT

Upper Respiratory Tract

Colds

MOST COMMON CAUSES   You've undoubtedly heard it hundreds of times, but since millions of colds are treated inappropriately every year, it bears repeating once more: *colds are caused by viruses, not bacteria*.

BEST TREATMENT   Your doctor knows the cause and treatment of colds and will be unlikely to prescribe antibiotics unless pressured, so don't ask for them.

Epiglottitis in adults

MOST COMMON CAUSES   Infection of the epiglottis, the flap of tissue that is the gateway to the vocal cords, is uncommon in adults and usually not too severe, but treatment should begin before the results of a throat culture are available. The most common causes are *Streptococcus* and *Hemophilus influenzae*.

BEST TREATMENT   The initial antibiotic should be the sulfa compound trimethoprim/sulfa, changed to penicillin if the culture demonstrates the cause is strep.

Epiglottitis in a child

MOST COMMON CAUSES   In contrast to adults, epiglottitis in children is a severe, life-threatening condition. The infection begins through the respiratory tract, and because of the marked inflammation of the epiglottis and the surrounding tissues, it may cause sudden respiratory obstruction. The distinguishing signs are a high fever, hoarseness, difficulty breathing and the characteristic barking cough, which differentiates it from the much milder croup. Croup is almost always caused by a virus, whereas epiglottitis is almost always caused by the bacterium *Hemophilus influenzae*.

BEST TREATMENT   Speed is vital. *The child with these symptoms should be taken to the emergency room immediately*. Besides making sure that the airway is open, intravenous antibiotic treatment with a third-generation cephalosporin such as ceftriaxone or cefotaxime should begin immediately.

Pharyngitis (tonsillitis)

MOST COMMON CAUSES   If pus is present on the tonsils and the patient has a fever, the disease is usually bacterial in origin. Although streptococci are the most common cause at any age, in sexually active adults occasionally the gonorrhea bacterium can be responsible.

BEST TREATMENT   A throat culture should be taken right away, unless the patient is extremely ill, and the best course is to wait until the results of the culture are available before beginning antibiotics. Besides, of course, allowing for the most specific treatment, there is growing evidence that waiting a day or two allows the body's immune defenses to help subdue the bacteria, and then the antibiotics can finish the job. Giving antibiotics right away may suppress the immune system.

When antibiotics are given, if the cause is strep, penicillin is still the recommended treatment, although in the past few years it has been documented that there are about 30 percent treatment failures with penicillin. This means that there is either a recurrence of the tonsillitis within three months or a repeat throat culture after the treatment shows the bacteria have not been eradicated. This is especially worrisome in children, since the main goal of treating pharyngitis in this age group is to prevent later development of rheumatic fever. In treatment failures, many experts now recommend treating with the first-generation cephalosporin cefadroxil. If the patient is allergic to penicillin, there are usually cross-allergies to cephalo-sporins, so erythromycin, azithromycin or clarithromycin is the choice. For a gonorrheal cause, a third-generation cephalosporin is the best antibiotic.

Laryngitis

MOST COMMON CAUSE   Almost always viral in origin.

BEST TREATMENT   No antibiotics indicated.

Acute Sinusitis

MOST COMMON CAUSES   Sinusitis can be caused by bacteria, viruses, fungi or allergic reactions, but an acute attack is usually a bacterial infection. Depending on what sinuses are involved, the common symptoms are headache or toothache, tenderness when the sinuses are touched. Fever is rarely present; when it is, it suggests some-thing more serious, such as an extension into the brain—a meningi-tis. Besides these signs, x-rays demonstrate an inflammation, and there is frequently a discharge through the nose that should be cul-tured. The most common bacteria found are streptococci, pneumo-cocci, staphylococci and, less commonly, *Hemophilus influenzae*.

BEST TREATMENT   Assuming an uncomplicated case, penicillin or erythromycin (in cases of penicillin allergy) should be started until the culture results are back. If the results indicate a staph or *Hemo-philus*, therapy can be changed to methicillin, ampicillin, or one of the newer erythromycins.

Chronic sinusitis (adult)

MOST COMMON CAUSES   More often anaerobic bacteria, including peptostreptococci, *Bacteroides* and *Fusobacterium*.

BEST TREATMENT   Metronidazole is effective against all possible bac-teria.

Chronic sinusitis (child)

MOST COMMON CAUSES   In children, chronic sinus infections are generally not caused by anaerobic bacteria. More likely, they will be due to pneumococcus, *Hemophilus* or another gram-negative bacteria called *Moraxella*.

BEST TREATMENT   The child should be started with the antibiotic trimethoprim/sulfa, which is generally effective against all the responsible bacteria. With chronic infections, it is not always possible to obtain material for culture. If the doctor is successful, therapy can be changed when the results are available. If, for example, the cause turns out to be pneumococcus, the antibiotic should be switched to penicillin.

LOWER RESPIRATORY TRACT

Acute bronchitis

MOST COMMON CAUSES   This condition is an acute inflammation of the bronchial passages. It is usually mild and self-limited, and most commonly caused by viruses, frequently following a cold. If there is fever or a pus-filled sputum present, a bacterial cause should be considered, the most likely of which are pneumococcus, *Chlamydia*, *Mycoplasma* or *Hemophilus*.

BEST TREATMENT   Unless the condition is thought to be bacterial, rest and aspirin or acetaminophen are the only treatment necessary. Otherwise, a sputum culture should be taken, and the patient started on azithromycin to cover all bacteria. When the culture report is available, the therapy can be shifted to penicillin if the cause was pneumococcus or to amoxicillin if the cause was a sensitive *Hemophilus*.

Bronchitis in children under five years old

MOST COMMON CAUSES   In almost all cases, this condition is caused by viruses.

BEST TREATMENT   Unless associated with an ear infection or a bacterial lung infection, no antibiotic treatment is called for.

Chronic bronchitis, acute bacterial exacerbation

MOST COMMON CAUSES   This is a condition of adults, and almost always occurs in smokers. Fever is rarely present, and often the only sign that there has been a recent bacterial infection is an increase in the daily production of sputum and a change in color from clear or yellow to green. In most cases, the responsible bacteria will be *Hemophilus, Moraxella* or pneumococcus.

BEST TREATMENT   A Gram stain of the sputum will usually show a mixture of bacteria and therefore not be of much help to the doctor in deciding the cause. Usually it will be necessary to wait for the culture. In the meantime, the one antibiotic that will reasonably cover all possibilities is trimethoprim/sulfa, which can be adjusted if need be when the culture and sensitivity tests are available.

Cystic fibrosis

MOST COMMON CAUSES   Patients with cystic fibrosis frequently get lung infections. In virtually all cases, they will be caused by some species of *Pseudomonas*.

BEST TREATMENT   Ciprofloxacin is quite effective against all species of *Pseudomonas*. This is a perfect example of why these newer antibiotics should be saved for diseases where they have special usefulness and why they shouldn't be used to treat conditions for which other antibiotics are effective.

Pneumonia

Although we tend to think of this as an infection of the past, it still affects some two million people annually in the United States, is the sixth leading cause of death overall and the most lethal of hospital-acquired infections. Pneumonia, an infection of the lungs, is caused by a wide range of microorganisms, depending mostly on age and underlying conditions. It is often extremely difficult to identify the responsible agent. Even though the doctor may have a clinical impression that the patient has pneumonia, in 30 to 50 percent of patients no specific pathogen is identifiable. Sputum specimens are often misleading owing to contamination by the normal bacterial population of the upper airways. In many patients, bacteria will be shed into the bloodstream, so blood cultures can sometimes be used to identify the causative organisms. In other cases material can be obtained by aspirating fluid for culture directly from the lower airways, inserting a needle either through the trachea or through the chest wall into the lungs. This, however, is obviously not a simple procedure and often patients with pneumonia are treated through the entire course of their disease without the specific bacterium being recognized. Fortunately, the physician does usually have some indirect evidence as a guideline to therapy, such as the clinical history, the pattern on x-ray and blood tests for antibodies.

Pneumonia in adults over thirty-five

MOST COMMON CAUSES   *Streptococcus pneumoniae*, or pneumococcus, is the most common cause of bacterial pneumonia that is not acquired in the hospital. It is a serious disease with a characteristically high fever, as well as distinctive x-ray, blood test and physical findings. A Gram stain and/or a culture of the sputum may demonstrate the bacteria, as may a blood culture. If there is an underlying chronic bronchitis, and the patient is not terribly sick, the next most likely cause is *Hemophilus influenzae*.

BEST TREATMENT   Unless there are some predisposing factors (see the other types of pneumonia) that could make another type of bacterium a more likely cause, these patients should be treated as if pneumococcus is the cause of their disease. It should always be considered serious and treated with high-dose penicillin until cultures indicate otherwise or there is no improvement after a couple of days. Although most strains of pneumococcus are still sensitive to penicillin, there has been a disturbing increase in resistant bacteria. In those cases, vancomycin may have to be used. If the cause is thought to be, or is identified as, *Hemophilus*, amoxicillin is usually effective, but may have to be changed to a cephalosporin when culture results are available.

Pneumonia in patients from five to thirty-five years old

MOST COMMON CAUSES   *Mycoplasma pneumoniae* is the most likely offender in this age group, followed by *Chlamydia pneumoniae*, a relative of the bacterium responsible for a great deal of sexually transmitted disease. Unlike pneumococcal pneumonia, which can come on suddenly, pneumonia due to these bacteria comes on and goes away gradually. This is not nearly as serious a condition as pneumococcal pneumonia. Patients rarely have to be hospitalized and almost always recover.

BEST TREATMENT   Erythromycin or one of its newer relatives, clarithromycin or azithromycin. The advantage of these newer antibiotics is that they don't upset the stomach nearly as much as erythromycin and have to be taken for only five days instead of the two- to three-week course recommended for erythromycin. The disadvantage is that they are more expensive, and being new agents, we want to preserve them as much as possible for more serious diseases.

Pneumonia in hospitalized elderly patients or patients in nursing homes

MOST COMMON CAUSES   In about 15 percent of the cases, *Staphylococcus* is the cause. In the others, the likely bacteria are gram-negative organisms such as *Klebsiella, Pseudomonas* and *Serratia*.

BEST TREATMENT   This is one of the cases in which it is difficult to sort out the cause of the disease from a contaminant of the upper airway. A culture of fluid aspirated directly from the respiratory tract is often indicated. But before culture results are available, a heavy antibiotic regimen must be started. The best choices to cover all possibilities and narrow selection for resistant bacteria include vancomycin, since 30 to 40 percent of nosocomial staphylococcal pneumonias are resistant to methicillin, and aztreonam, an injectable antibiotic that is active only against gram-negative bacteria. Aztreonam has a spectrum of activity similar to gentamicin and tobramycin's, but is less toxic to the kidneys, frequently an important consideration in debilitated elderly people whose kidney function may already be diminished.

Pneumonia in an infant or intravenous drug abuser

MOST COMMON CAUSES   For different reasons, the immune systems of infants and drug abusers function as poorly as those of the elderly and thus they are susceptible to the same organisms: staphylococci and gram-negative bacteria, the same bacteria that cause pneumonia in the elderly.

BEST TREATMENT   Vancomycin and aztreonam, gentamicin or tobramycin (in much smaller doses for infants), until the culture results are ready.

SKIN

Acne vulgaris

MOST COMMON CAUSES   Acne is not a skin infection, although the pimples (technically called comedones) can become infected. In the past, it was common to treat any patient who had acne with a daily dose of tetracycline, whether or not a skin infection was present. It is this sort of irrational policy that has helped propagate and perpetuate antibiotic resistance. Fortunately this regimen is not often followed today, mostly because of the availability of topical and systemic vitamin A–like compounds (Retin-A and Accutane) which have proven remarkably effective in treating mild and severe acne respectively. When an infection does occur, the most common organism involved is the bacterium called *Propionibacterium acnes*.

BEST TREATMENT   Topical clindamycin should be tried first. If that is ineffective, the next choice should be erythromycin and finally the broad-spectrum tetracycline.

Burns

MOST COMMON CAUSES   Once a burn has occurred and the integrity of the skin broken, there is an open portal of entry for bacteria. Combined with the suppression of the immune system that accompanies burns, it is a perfect setup for infections. We should emphasize that we are talking about second- or third-degree burns that involve a significant amount of body surface area. In many cases, although not always, hospitalization will be required. The list of bacteria that could be involved is long and includes staphylococci (methicillin-sensitive and -resistant), streptococci, *Serratia*, Enterobacteriaceae and *Pseudomonas*.

BEST TREATMENT   Topical ointments of silver sulfadiazine are often used, in combination with a regimen of antibiotics including vancomycin, a third-generation cephalosporin and trimethoprim/sulfa. These are necessary to cover all bacterial possibilities. The treatment can and should be fine-tuned when burn culture results are available.

Impetigo

MOST COMMON CAUSES   This is a skin infection primarily of children, caused usually by streptococci but occasionally by staph.

BEST TREATMENT   Until cultures are available, both bacteria have to be accounted for. Methicillin-resistant staph sometimes cause impetigo, but this condition is not serious enough to warrant using vancomycin immediately. Either erythromycin or amoxicillin/clavulanic acid should be the initial choice.

Recurrent boils

MOST COMMON CAUSES   Boils are sometimes infected with bacteria, sometimes not. When bacteria are present, staphylococci, both methicillin-sensitive and -resistant, are the usual offenders.

BEST TREATMENT   For an acute episode, antibiotics are considered of questionable value. However, most experts recommend a course of antibiotic treatment with topical mupirocin instilled in the nose, along with an antistaphylococcal penicillin such as methicillin or dicloxacillin by mouth, in order to prevent recurrences.

III. Names and Addresses of Organizations and Individuals Concerned with Proper Antibiotic Use

Alliance for the Prudent Use of Antibiotics, PO Box 1372, Boston, MA 02117-1372; 617-956-6765

American Association of Medical Colleges, 2450 N St. NW, Washington, DC 20037-1126; 202-828-0400; Donald G. Kassebaum, M.D., Associate Secretary

American Medical Association, 515 N. State St., Chicago, IL 60610; 312-464-5000; James S. Todd, M.D., Exec. Vice President

American Veterinary Medical Association, 930 Meacham Rd., Schaumberg, IL 60196; 708-605-8070; Michael Walters, DVM, Public Information Director

Dr. Jerry Avorn, Professor of Social Medicine and Health Policy, Harvard Medical School, 221 Longwood Ave., Boston, MA 02115; 617-278-0930

Food Animals Concern Trust (FACT), PO Box 14599, Chicago, IL 60614; 312-525-4952

Joint Commission on the Accreditation of Healthcare Organizations, One Renaissance Blvd., Oakbrook Terrace, IL 60181; 708-916-5600; Dennis S. O'Leary, M.D., President

Mr. Don Kitajima, Kaiser Regional Pharmacy, 1800 Harrison St., Oakland, CA 94302; 510-987-2408

Mr. Terry Latanich, Senior Vice President, Medco Containment Services, Inc., 100 Summit Ave., Montvale, NJ 07645; 201-358-5400

Dr. Philip Lee, Assistant Secretary, Department of Health and Human Services, 200 Independence Ave. SW, Washington, DC 20201; 202-690-8157

Liaison Committee on Medical Education, 515 N. State St., Chicago, IL 60610; 312-464-4657; Harry Jonas, M.D., Secretary

MacroMed, 13025 Bailey St., Suite D, Whittier, CA 90601; 800-848-8726

National Cattlemen's Association, PO Box 3469, Englewood, CO 80155; 303-694-0305; Earl Peterson, Exec. Vice President

National Institutes of Health, 9000 Rockville Pike, Bethesda, MD 20892; 301-496-4000

National Pork Producers Council, PO Box 10383, Des Moines, IA 50306; 515-223-2600; Russ Sanders, Exec. Vice President

Natural Resources Defense Council, 40 W. 20th St., New York, NY 10011; 212-727-4400

Poultry Science Association, 309 W. Clark St., Champaign, IL 61820; 217-356-3182; C.D. Johnson, Business Manager
(Poultry breeding is overseen regionally, so it's best to contact this organization, which is engaged in teaching and technical services for the poultry industry.)

World Health Organization, Avenue Appia 11, Geneva 27, Switzerland

For the addresses of your local and state medical societies, contact them directly by telephone.

Acknowledgments

I am deeply indebted to several researchers and clinicians who shared with me their scientific insights and their time as I was developing this book. I am especially grateful to two of them. Dr. Thomas O'Brien, medical director of the microbiology lab at Brigham and Women's Hospital in Boston and associate professor of medicine at Harvard Medical School, not only provided me with valuable information, but also shared with me in great detail the operation of the busy, state-of-the-art laboratory he oversees in Boston.

Professor Luc Montagnier of the Institut Pasteur in Paris was more than generous with his time in September 1992, immediately after he had revealed his elegant and still somewhat controversial theory about AIDS at the International AIDS Convention in Amsterdam. Knowing how besieged Dr. Montagnier was by the media and the scientific community to give interviews and make personal appearances, I appreciate his professional disclosures all the more.

The other physicians whom I thank are (in alphabetical order):

Dr. Jerry Avorn, Professor of Social Medicine and Health Policy, Harvard University School of Medicine

Dr. Mitchell Cohen, Chief, Division of Bacterial Infections, Centers for Disease Control and Prevention

Dr. Peter Duesberg, Professor, Department of Molecular Biology, University of California, Berkeley

Dr. Harry Gallis, Department of Medicine, Division of Infectious Diseases, Duke University School of Medicine

Dr. Donald Kollisch, Family Practice Program, University of North Carolina School of Medicine

Dr. Calvin Kunin, Chief of Infectious Diseases, Department of Medicine, Ohio State University School of Medicine

Dr. Stuart Levy, Departments of Microbiology and Molecular Biology, Tufts University School of Medicine

Dr. Daniel Musher, Chief of Infectious Diseases, Department of Medicine, Baylor University School of Medicine

Dr. Robert S. Root-Bernstein, Associate Professor, Department of Physiology, Michigan State University

Dr. David Shlaes, Division of Infectious Diseases, Department of Medicine, Case Western Reserve University School of Medicine

Dr. Richard Wenzel, Chief of Infectious Diseases, University of Iowa School of Medicine

Dr. Shyh-Ching Lo, Chief, Division of Molecular Pathology, Armed Forces Institute of Pathology

Dr. Victor Yu, Division of Infectious Diseases, Department of Medicine, University of Pittsburgh School of Medicine

Besides scientific help, I have received invaluable assistance from several other sources. Once again Fred Hills, my editor at Simon & Schuster, immediately grasped the significance of *The Plague Makers* and served as a champion and guiding force throughout. I am also grateful to his extremely capable and experienced associate, Burton Beals, for editorial comments and direction. David Anderson provided editorial assistance in the early chapters and I thank him as well.

Then there is my core group of support without whose astuteness and forbearance neither this nor any other project I attempt would be completed. My agents, Herb and Nancy Katz, as usual, provided direction, encouragement and wisdom far beyond what I had any right to expect. Finally, my wife, Liz, was there for me always, with a kind word and an often much-needed hug. With each succeeding book, I love and respect her more.

Bibliography

CHAPTER 1. PRELUDE TO DISASTER

Appelbaum PC. Antimicrobial resistance in *Streptococcus pneumoniae*: an overview. *Clinical Infectious Diseases* 1992; 15:77–83.

Appelbaum PC, Scragg JN, Bowen AJ, et al. *Streptococcus pneumoniae* resistant to penicillin and chloramphenicol. *Lancet* 1977; 2:995–97.

Barber M, Dutton AAC. Antibiotic-resistant staphylococcal outbreaks in a medical and a surgical ward. *Lancet* 1958; 1:64–68.

Bennett PM, Hawkey PM. The future contribution of transposition to antimicrobial resistance. *Journal of Hospital Infection* 1991; 18:211–21.

Buu-Hoi A, Horodniceanu B. Conjugative transfer of multiple antibiotic resistance markers in *Streptococcus pneumoniae*. *Journal of Bacteriology* 1980; 143:313–20.

Casewell MW, Talsania HG, Knight S. Gentamicin-resistant *Klebsiella aerogenes* as a clinically significant source of transferable antibiotic resistance. *Journal of Antimicrobial Chemotherapy* 1981; 8:153–60.

Chopra I. Antibiotic resistance resulting from decreased drug accumulation. *British Medical Bulletin* 1984:11–17.

Cohen ML. Epidemiology of drug resistance: implications for a postantimicrobial era. *Science* 1992; 257:1050–54.

Echeverria P, Ulyangco CV, Ho MT. Antimicrobial resistance and enterotoxin production among isolates of *Escherichia coli* in the Far East. *Lancet* 1978 1:589–92.

Eickhoff TC, Finland M. Changing susceptibility of meningococci to antimicrobial agents. *New England Journal of Medicine* 1962; 272(8):395–97.

Farrar WE. Antibiotic resistance in bacteria: mechanisms and consequences. *Emory University Journal of Medicine* 1990; 4:229–36.

Finland M. Changing patterns of susceptibility of common bacterial pathogens to antimicrobial agents. *Annals of Internal Medicine* 1972; 76:1009–36.

Finland M. And the walls come tumbling down. *New England Journal of Medicine* 1978; 299:770–71.

Goodier TEW, Parry WR. Sensitivity of clinically important bacteria to six common antibacterial substances. *Lancet* 1959; 1:356–57.

Hamilton-Miller JMT. The emergence of antibiotic resistance: myths and facts in clinical practice. *Intensive Care Medicine* 1990; 16:s206–11.

Hawkey PM. Resistant bacteria in the normal human flora. *Journal of Antimicrobial Chemotherapy* 1986; 18(supplement C):133–39.

Hughes VM, Datta N. Conjugative plasmids in bacteria of the "pre-antibiotic" era. *Nature* 1983; 302:725–26.

Hummel RP, Miskell PW, Altemeier WA. Antibiotic resistance transfer from non-pathogenic to pathogenic bacteria. *Surgery* 1977; 82(3):382–85.

Iannini PB, Eickhoff TC, Laforce FM. Multidrug-resistant *Proteus rettgeri*: an emerging problem. *Annals of Internal Medicine* 1976; 85:161–64.

Jacobs MR, Koornhof HJ, Robins-Browne RM, et al. Emergence of multiply resistant pneumococci. *New England Journal of Medicine* 1978; 299:735–40.

Krause RM. The origin of plagues: old and new. *Science* 1992; 257:1073–76.

Lambert HP. Impact of bacterial resistance to antibiotics on therapy. *British Medical Bulletin* 1984; 40:102–6.

Levy SB. Microbial resistance to antibiotics: an evolving and persistent problem. *Lancet* 1982; 1:83–88.

Levy SB. Starting life resistance-free. *New England Journal of Medicine* 1990; 323:335–36.

Levy SB. Antibiotic availability and use: consequences to man and his environment. *Journal of Clinical Epidemiology* 1991; 44:83s–87s.

Levy SB, Marshall B, Schluederberg S. High frequency of antimicrobial resistance in human fecal flora. *Antimicrobial Agents and Chemotherapy* 1988; 32(12):1801–6.

Marks MI. *Hemophilus influenzae* infections. *Clinical Pediatrics* 1984; 23:535–41.

Medeiros AA. Beta-lactamases. *British Medical Bulletin* 1984; 40:18–27.

Murray BE. New aspects of antimicrobial resistance and the resulting therapeutic dilemmas. *Journal of Infectious Diseases* 1993; 163:1185–94.

Neu HC. The crisis in antibiotic resistance. *Science* 1992; 257:1064–73.

O'Brien TF, and members of the task force 2. Resistance of bacteria to antibacterial agents: report of task force 2. *Reviews of Infectious Diseases* 1987: 9(supplement 3):s244–60.

O'Brien TF, Mayer KH, Kishi H, et al. Intercontinental spread of a new antibiotic resistance gene on an epidemic plasmid. *Science* 1985; 320:87–89.

Pollock AV, Evans M. Changing patterns of bacterial resistance in relation to prophylactic use of cephaloridine and therapeutic use of ampicillin. *Lancet* 1975; 2:1251–54.

Reynolds PE. Resistance of the antibiotic target site. *British Medical Bulletin* 1984; 40:3–10.

Saunders JR. Genetics and evolution of antibiotic resistance. *British Medical Bulletin* 1984; 40:54–60.

Seppala H, Nissinen A, Jarvinen H, et al. Resistance to erythromycin in group A streptococci. *New England Journal of Medicine* 1992; 326:292–97.

Shafran SD. The basis of antibiotic resistance in bacteria. *Journal of Otolaryngology* 1990; 19:158–68.

Stollerman GH. Trends in bacterial virulence and antibiotic susceptibility: strepto-cocci, pneumococci and gonococci. *Annals of Internal Medicine* 1978; 89:746–48.

Syriopoulou V, Scheifele D, Smith AL, et al. Increasing incidence of ampicillin resis-tance in *Hemophilus influenzae. Journal of Pediatrics* 1978; 92(6):889–92.

Watanabe T. Infectious drug resistance. *Scientific American* 1967; 217(6):19–27.

Woolfrey BF, Lally RT, Ireland GK, et al. Antimicrobial resistance in *Hemophilus* iso-lates: a Minnesota experience and literature review. *American Journal of Clinical Pathology* 1984; 82:311–18.

Chapter 2. Hospitals: The Places You Go to Get Sick

Barrett FF, Casey JI, Finland M. Infections and antibiotic use among patients at Bos-ton City Hospital, February, 1967. *New England Journal of Medicine* 1968; 278:5–9.

Barriere SL, Conte JE. Emergence of multiple antibiotic resistance during the therapy of *Klebsiella pneumoniae* meningitis. *American Journal of the Medical Sciences* 1980; 279:61–64.

Brumfitt W, Hamilton-Miller J. Methicillin-resistant *Staphylococcus aureus. New En-gland Journal of Medicine* 1989; 320:1188–96.

Chow JW, Fine MJ, Shlaes DM. *Enterobacter* bacteremia: clinical features and emer-gence of antibiotic resistance during therapy. *Annals of Internal Medicine* 1991; 115:585–90.

Classen DC, Evans RS, Pestotnik SL. The timing of prophylactic administration of antibiotics and the risk of surgical-wound infection. *New England Journal of Med-icine* 1992; 326:281–86.

Constantine LM, Scott S. Inappropriate use of antibiotics and the rise of resistant or-ganisms. *American Pharmacy* 1991; 271:23–25.

Dlan HF, Morgan AF, Asche V, et al. Isolates of *Pseudomonas aeruginosa* from Aus-tralian hospitals having R-plasmid determined antibiotic resistance. *Medical Jour-nal of Australia* 1977; 2:116–19.

Finland M. Superinfections in the antibiotic era. *Postgraduate Medicine* 1973; 54:175–82.

Friedan TR, Mangi RJ. Inappropriate use of oral ciprofloxacin. *Journal of the Ameri-can Medical Association* 1990; 264:1438–40.

Hamilton-Miller JMT. Use and abuse of antibiotics. *British Journal of Clinical Phar-macology* 1984; 18:469–74.

Handwerger S, Perlman DC, Altarac D, McAuliffe V. Concomitant high-level vanco-mycin and penicillin resistance in clinical isolates of enterococci. *Clinical Infectious Diseases* 1992; 14:655–61.

Kunin C, Efron HY. Audits of antimicrobial usage. *Journal of the American Medical Association* 1977; 237:1001–2.

Kunin C, Tupasi T, Craig W. Misuse of antibiotics. *Annals of Internal Medicine* 1973; 79:555–60.

Maki DG, Schuna AA. A study of antimicrobial misuse in a university hospital. *Amer-ican Journal of the Medical Sciences* 1978; 275:271–81.

Mouton RP, Glerum JH, Loenen AC. Relationship between antibiotic consumption and frequency of antibiotic resistance of four pathogens—a seven-year survey. *Journal of Antimicrobial Chemotherapy* 1976; 2:9–19.

Muder RR, Brennen C, Waegner MM. Methicillin-resistant staphylococci colonization and infection in a long-term care facility. *Annals of Internal Medicine* 1991; 114:107–12.

Mylotte JM. Gentamicin resistance among gram-negative bacillary blood isolates in a hospital with long-term use of gentamicin. *Archives of Internal Medicine* 1987; 147:1642–44.

Nachamkin J, Axelrod P, Talbot S., et al. Multiply high-level aminoglycoside resistant enterococci isolated from patients in a university hospital. *Journal of Clinical Microbiology* 1988; 26:1287–91.

Raviglione MC, Boyle JF, Mariuz P, et al. Ciprofloxacin-resistant methicillin-resistant *Staphylococus aureus* in an acute care hospital. *Antimicrobial Agents and Chemotherapy* 1990; 34:2050–54.

Richmond AS, Rahal JJ, Simberkoff MS, Schlaeffer S. R factors in gentamicin-resistant organisms causing hospital infection. *Lancet* 1975; 2:1176–78.

Schaberg DR, Alford RH, Anderson R, et al. An outbreak of nosocomial infection due to multiply resistant *Serratia marcescens:* evidence of interhospital spread. *Journal of Infectious Diseases* 1976; 134:181–88.

Schaberg DR, Culver DH, Gaynes RP. Major trends in the microbial etiology of nosocomial infection. *American Journal of Medicine* 1991; 91:72s–75s.

Schaffner W, Ray WA, Federspiel CF. Surveillance of antibiotic prescribing in office practice. *Annals of Internal Medicine* 1978; 89:796–99.

Shlaes DM, Bouvet A, Devine C, et al. Inducible, transferable resistance to vancomycin in *Enterococcus faecalis* A256. *Antimicrobial Agents and Chemotherapy* 1989; 33:198–203.

Siebert WT, Moreland NJ, Williams TW. Resistance to gentamicin: a growing concern. *Southern Medical Journal* 1977; 70:289–92.

Simmons HE, Stolley PD. This is medical progress? Trends and consequences of antibiotic use in the United States. *Journal of the American Medical Association* 1974; 227:1023–32.

Sugarman B, Pesanti E. Treatment failures secondary to in vivo development of drug resistance by microorganisms. *Reviews of Infectious Diseases* 1980; 2:153–68.

Swindell PJ, Reeves DS, Bullock DW, et al. Audits of antibiotic prescribing in a Bristol hospital. *British Medical Journal* 1983; 286:118–22.

Thomas FE, Jackson RT, Melly A, Alford RH. Sequential hospitalwide outbreaks of resistant *Serratia* and *Klebsiella* infections. *Archives of Internal Medicine* 1977; 137:581–84.

Vincent S, Minkler P, Bincziewski B, et al. Vancomycin resistance in *Enterococcus gallinarum*. *Antimicrobial Agents and Chemotherapy* 1992; 36:1392–95.

Chapter 3. Apocalypse Soon?

Beck-Sagué C, Dooley SW, Hutton MD, et al. Hospital outbreak of multidrug-resistant *Mycobacterium tuberculosis* infections: factors in transmission to staff and HIV-infected patients. *Journal of the American Medical Association* 1992; 268:1280–86.

Bellin EY, Fletcher DD, Safyer SM. Association of tuberculosis infection with increased time in or admission to the New York City jail system. *Journal of the American Medical Association* 1993; 269:2228–31.

Bloom BR. Back to a frightening future. *Nature* 1992; 358:538–39.

Bloom BR. Testimony before Human Resources and Intergovernmental Relations Subcommittee, Committee on Government Operations, US House of Representatives, April 2, 1992.

Bloom BR, Murray CJL. Tuberculosis: commentary on a reemergent killer. *Science* 1992; 257:1055–63.

Chawla PK, Klapper PJ, Kamholz SL, et al. Drug resistant tuberculosis in an urban population including patients at risk for human immunodeficiency virus infection. *American Review of Respiratory Diseases* 1992; 146:280–84.

Dooley SW, Jarvis WR, Martone WJ, Snider DE. Multidrug-resistant tuberculosis. *Annals of Internal Medicine* 1992; 117:257–58.

Fauci AS. Statement before the Human Resources and Intergovernmental Relations Subcommittee, Committee on Government Operations, US House of Representatives, April 2, 1992.

Fischl MA, Daikos GL, Uttamchandani RB, et al. Clinical presentation and outcome of patients with HIV infection and tuberculosis caused by multiple-drug-resistant bacilli. *Annals of Internal Medicine* 1992; 117:184–90.

Fischl MA, Uttamchandani RB, Daikos GL, et al. An outbreak of tuberculosis caused by multiple-drug-resistant tuberculosis among patients with HIV infection. *Annals of Internal Medicine* 1992; 117:177–83.

Glassworth J. Tuberculosis in the United States: looking for a silver lining among the clouds. *American Review of Respiratory Diseases* 1992; 146:278–79.

Mitchison DA. Drug resistance in Mycobacteria. *British Medical Bulletin* 1984; 40:84–90.

Roper W. Statement before the Human Resources and Intergovernmental Relations Subcommittee, Committee on Government Operations, US House of Representatives, April 2, 1992.

Zhang Y, Heym, Allen B, et al. The catalase-peroxidase gene and isoniazid resistance of *Mycobacterium tuberculosis*. *Nature* 1992; 358:591–93.

Chapter 4. The Possible Link Between Antibiotics and AIDS

and

Chapter 5. Completing the AIDS Hypothesis

Beach RS, Mantero-Atienza E, Shor-Posner G, et al. Specific nutrient abnormalities in asymptomatic HIV-1 infection. *AIDS* 1992; 6:701–7.

Branbilla G. Genotoxic effects of drug/nitrite interaction products: evidence for the need of risk assessment. *Pharmacological Research Communications* 1985; 17:307–19.

Chandra RK. Single nutrient deficiency and cell-mediated immune responses. *American Journal of Clinical Nutrition* 1980; 33:736–38.

Christiansson A, Mardh P. Tetracycline resistance in *Mycoplasma hominis. Sexually Transmitted Diseases* 1983; 11:371–73.

Della Bovi P, Donti E, Knowles DM, et al. Presences of chromosomal abnormalities and lack of retrovirus DNA sequences in AIDS-associated Kaposi's sarcoma. *Cancer Research* 1986; 46:6333–38.

Duesberg PH. Retroviruses as carcinogens and pathogens: expectations and reality. *Cancer Research* 1987; 47:1199–1220.

Duesberg PH. AIDS epidemiology: inconsistencies with human immunodeficiency virus and with infectious disease. *Proceedings of the National Academy of Sciences USA* 1991; 88:1575–79.

Editorial. Mycoplasma and AIDS—what connection? *Lancet* 1991; 337:20–21.

Goldsmith M. Science ponders whether HIV acts alone or has another microbe's aid. *Journal of the American Medical Association* 1990; 264:665–66.

Goldsmith M. Still a mystery but "not likely" a virus. *Journal of the American Medical Association* 1992; 258:1235–45.

Grinspoon SK, Bilezikian JP. HIV disease and the endocrine system. *New England Journal of Medicine* 1992; 327:1360–65.

Haverkos HW, Pinsky PF, Drotman P, Bregman DJ. Disease manifestation among homosexual men with acquired immunodeficiency syndrome: a possible role of nitrites in Kaposi's sarcoma. *Sexually Transmitted Diseases* 1985; 13:203–8.

Jaffe HW, Keewhan C, Thomas PA, et al. National case-control study of Kaposi's sarcoma and *Pneumocystis carinii* pneumonia in homosexual men; part I, epidemiologic results. *Annals of Internal Medicine* 1983; 99:145–51.

Krause, R. The origin of plagues: old and new. *Science* 1992; 257:1073–77.

Lemaitre M, Henin Y, Destouesse F, Ferrieux C, Montagnier L, Blanchard A. Role of *Mycoplasma* infection in the cytopathic effect induced by human immunodeficiency virus type I in infected cell lines. *Infection and Immunity* 1992; 60:742–48.

Lo S-C. A newly identified human *Mycoplasma* disease. *Infectious Disease Newsletter* 1990; 9:73–76.

Lo S-C. Enhancement of HIV-i cytocidal effects in CD4+ lymphocytes by the AIDS-associated *Mycoplasma. Science* 1991; 251:1074–76.

Lo S-C. *Mycoplasma* infections in AIDS. *Virology* 1991; 143–45.

Lo S-C, Dawson MS, Newton PB, et al. Association of the virus-like infectious agent originally reported in patients with AIDS with acute fatal disease in previously healthy non-AIDS patients. *American Journal of Tropical Medicine and Hygiene* 1989; 41:364–76.

Lo S-C, Dawson MS, Wong DM, et al. Identification of *Mycoplasma incognitus* infection in patients with AIDS: an immunohistochemical, in situ hybridization and ultrastructural study. *American Journal of Tropical Medicine and Hygiene* 1989; 41:601–16.

Lo S-C, Hayes MM, Wang R, et al. Newly discovered *Mycoplasma* isolated from patients infected with HIV. *Lancet* 1991; 338:1415–18.

Lo S-C, Shih J, Yang N, et al. A novel virus-like infectious agent in patients with AIDS. *American Journal of Tropical Medicine and Hygiene* 1989; 40:213–26.

Lo S-C, Shih JW, Newton PB, et al. Virus-like infectious agent (VLIA) is a novel pathogenic *Mycoplasma: Mycoplasma incognitus. American Journal of Tropical Medicine and Hygiene* 1989; 41:586–600.

Lo S-C, Wang R, Newton P, et al. Fatal infection of silvered leaf monkeys with a virus-like infectious agent (VLIA) derived from a patient with AIDS. *American Journal of Tropical Medicine and Hygiene* 1989; 50:399–409.

Maddox, J. Rage and confusion hide role of HIV. *Nature* 1992; 357:188–89.

Miller GG, Strittmatter WJ. Identification of human T cells that require zinc for growth. *Scandinavian Journal of Immunology* 1992; 36:269–77.

Munster AM, Loadholdt B, Leary AG, Barnes MA. The effect of antibiotics on cell-mediated immunity. *Surgery* 1977; 81:692–95.

Osterloh J, Goldfield S. Butyl nitrite transformation in vitro, chemical nitrosation reactions and mutagenesis. *Journal of Analytical Toxicology* 1984; 8:164–68.

Pifer LL, Wang Y, Chiang TM, et al. Borderline immunodeficiency in male homosexuals: is life-style contributory? *Southern Medical Journal* 1987; 80:688–97.

Root-Bernstein, R. Do we know the causes of AIDS? *Perspectives in Biology and Medicine* 1990; 33:480–500.

Root-Bernstein, R. *Rethinking AIDS: The Tragic Cost of Premature Consensus.* The Free Press (New York), 1992.

Root-Bernstein, R. Rethinking AIDS. *Wall Street Journal;* April 17, 1993.

Roszkowski W, Ko HL, Roszkowski K, et al. Antibiotics and immunomodulation: effects of cefotaxime, amikacin, mezlocillin, piperacillin and clindamycin. *Medical Microbiology and Immunology* 1985; 173:279–89.

Saillard C, Carle P, Bove JM. Genetic and serologic relatedness between *Mycoplasma fermentans* strains and a *Mycoplasma* recently identified in tissues of AIDS and non-AIDS patients. *Research in Virology* 1990; 141:385–95.

Tarnawski A, Batko B. Antibiotics and immune processes. *Lancet* 1973; 1:674–75.

Wright K. Mycoplasmas in the AIDS spotlight. *Science* 1990; 248:682–83.

CHAPTER 6. DANGEROUS EXPORTS FROM THE THIRD WORLD

Ellis CJ. Antibiotic resistance in the tropics: the use of antibiotics in the tropics. *Transactions of the Royal Society of Tropical Medicine and Hygiene* 1989; 83:37–48.

Farrar WE. Antibiotic resistance in developing countries. *Journal of Infectious Diseases* 1985; 152:1103–06.

Geest S. The illegal distribution of Western medicines in developing countries: pharmacists, drug pedlars, injection doctors, and others. *Medical Anthropology;* Fall 1982:197–219.

Hossain MM, Glass RI, Khan MR. Antibiotic use in a rural community in Bangladesh. *International Journal of Epidemiology* 1982; 11:402–5.

Kunin CM. Antibiotic resistance: a world health problem we cannot ignore. *Annals of Internal Medicine* 1983; 99:859–60.

Kunin CM. Pharmacoepidemiology in developing countries. *Journal of Clinical Epidemiology* 1991; 44:1s–6s.

Kunin CM. Resistance to antimicrobial drugs—a worldwide calamity. *Annals of Internal Medicine* 1993; 118:557–60.

Lee PR, Lurie P, Silverman MM, Lydecker M. Drug promotion and labeling in developing countries: an update. *Journal of Clinical Epidemiology* 1991; 44 (supplement II):49s–55s.

Lester SC, Pla M, Wang F, et al. The carriage of *Escherichia coli* resistant to antimicrobial agents by healthy children in Boston, in Caracas, Venezuela and in Qin Pu, China. *New England Journal of Medicine* 1990; 323:285–89.

Melrose D. *Bitter Pills: Medicines and the Third World Poor.* Oxfam (Oxford), 1982.

Michel JM. Why do people like medicines? A perspective from Africa. *Lancet* 1985; 1:210–11.

Rudy RP, Murray BE. Evidence for an epidemic trimethoprim-resistance plasmid in fecal isolates of *Escherichia coli* from citizens of the United States studying in Mexico. *Journal of Infectious Diseases* 1984; 150:25–29.

Stein CM, Todd WTA, Parienyatwa D, Chakonda J, Dizwani AGM. A survey of antibiotic use in Harare primary care clinics. *Journal of Antimicrobial Chemotherapy* 1984; 14:149–56.

Thamlikitkul V. Antibiotic dispensing by drug store personnel in Bangkok, Thailand. *Journal of Antimicrobial Chemotherapy* 1988; 21:125–31.

World Health Organization. *The World Drug Situation.* Geneva, 1988.

CHAPTER 7. BIGGER ANIMALS, MORE RESISTANCE

Antibiotic resistance. Hearings before the Subcommittee on Investigations and Oversight of the Committee on Science and Technology, US House of Representatives. Ninety-eighth Congress, Second Session, December 18–19, 1984.

Corpet DE. Antibiotic residues and drug resistance in human intestinal flora. *Antimicrobial Agents and Chemotherapy* 1987; 31:587–93.

Hirsh DC, Ling GV, Ruby AL. Incidence of R-plasmids in fecal flora of healthy household dogs. *Antimicrobial Agents and Chemotherapy* 1980; 17:313–15.

Holmberg SD, et al. Drug resistant *Salmonella* from animals fed antibiotics. *New England Journal of Medicine* 1987; 311:617–22.

Institute of Medicine. *Human Health Risks with the Subtherapeutic Uses of Penicillin or Tetracyclines in Animal Feed.* National Academy Press (Washington), 1989.

Jukes TH. Public health significance of feeding low levels of antibiotics to animals. *Advances in Applied Microbiology* 1973; 16:1–29.

Jukes TH. Effects of low levels of antibiotics in livestock feeds. Presented at an American Chemical Society Symposium, Chicago, Illinois, September 8–13, 1985.

Lafont JP, Guillot JF, Chaslus-Danela E, et al. Antibiotic-resistant bacteria in animal wastes: a human health hazard? *Bulletin de L'Institut Pasteur* 1981; 79:213–31.

Levy SB. Antibiotic use for growth promotion in animals: ecologic and public health consequences. *Journal of Food Protection* 1987; 50:616–20.

Levy SB, Fitzgerald GG, Macone AB. Changes in the intestinal flora of farm personnel after introduction of tetracycline-supplemented feed on a farm. *New England Journal of Medicine* 1976; 295:583–88.

Linton AH. Antibiotic resistant bacteria in animal husbandry. *British Medical Bulletin* 1984; 40:91–95.

Linton AH. Flow of resistance genes in the environment and from animals to man. *Journal of Antimicrobial Chemotherapy* 1986; 18(supplement C):189–97.

Remington JS, Schimpff SC. Please don't eat the salads. *New England Journal of Medicine* 1981; 304:433–34.

Spika JS, Waterman SH, Soo Hoo GW, et al. Chloramphenicol-resistant *Salmonella newport* traced through hamburger to dairy farms. *New England Journal of Medicine* 1987; 316:565–80.

Chapter 8. First Cures, First Problems

and

Chapter 9. More Cures and the Widening Problem

Abraham EP, Chain E. An enzyme from bacteria able to destroy penicillin. *Nature* 1940; 3713:837.

Carithers HA. The first use of an antibiotic in America. *American Journal of Diseases of Children* 1974; 128:207–11.

Comroe JH. Pay dirt: the story of streptomycin. *American Review of Respiratory Disease* 1978; 117:773–80.

Fleming A. On the antibacterial action of cultures of a *Penicillium*, with special reference to their use in the isolation of *B. influenzae*. *British Journal of Experimental Pathology* 1929; 10:226–36.

Hare R. *The Birth of Penicillin and the Disarming of the Microbes*. George Allen and Unwin (London), 1975.

Hare R. New light on the history of penicillin. *Medical History* 1982; 26:1–24.

Hirsch JG. The greatest success story in the history of medicine. *Medical Times* 1980; 108:36–43.

MacFarlane G. *Alexander Fleming: The Man and the Myth*. Chatto and Windus (London), 1984.

Masters D. *Miracle Drug: The Inner History of Penicillin*. Eyre and Spottiswoode (London), 1946.

Wainwright M. The history of the therapeutic use of crude penicillin. *Medical History* 1987; 31:41–50.

Wainwright, M. Selman Waksman and the streptomycin controversy. *Society of Microbiology General Quarterly* 1988; 15:90–92.

Wainwright M. *Miracle Cure: The Story of Penicillin and the Golden Age of Antibiotics*. Blackwell (Oxford), 1990.

Waksman SA. *My Life with the Microbes*. Simon & Schuster (New York), 1954.

Williams TI. *Howard Florey: Penicillin and After*. Oxford University Press (Oxford), 1984.

Woodruff HB, Bury RW. The antibiotic explosion. *Discoveries in Pharmacology* 1986; 3:303–51.

CHAPTER 10. THE MISEDUCATION OF PHYSICIANS

Advertising, marketing and promotional practices of the pharmaceutical industry. Hearing before the Committee on Labor and Human Resources, US Senate. One hundred first Congress, Second Session, December 11–12, 1990.

Avorn J, Chen M, Hartley R. Scientific versus commercial sources of influence on the prescribing behavior of physicians. *American Journal of Medicine* 1982; 73:4–8.

Bero LA, Galbraith A, Rennie D. The publication of sponsored symposiums in medical journals. *New England Journal of Medicine* 1992; 327:1135–40.

Cooke D, Salter AJ, Phillips I. Antimicrobial misuse, antibiotic policies and information resources. *Journal of Antimicrobial Chemotherapy* 1980; 6:435–43.

Dajda R. Drug advertising and prescribing. *Journal of the Royal College of Physicians* 1978; 28:538–41.

Goldberg R. The myth of high cost drugs. *Wall Street Journal*, September 29, 1992.

Goldstein J. Of mugs and marketing. *Journal of the American Medical Association* 1991; 265:2391–92.

Haynes RB, Davis DA, McKibbon A, Tugwell P. A critical appraisal of the efficacy of continuing medical education. *Journal of the American Medical Association* 1984; 251:61–64.

Hemminki E. Review of the literature of the factors affecting drug prescribing. *Social Science and Medicine* 1974; 9:111–15.

Hemminki E. Content analysis of drug-detailing by pharmaceutical representatives. *Medical Education* 1977; 11:210–15.

Kim JH, Gallis HA. Observations on spiraling empiricism: its causes, allure and perils, with particular reference to antibiotic therapy. *American Journal of Medicine* 1989; 87:201–5.

Kunin CM. The responsibility of the infectious disease community for the optimal use of antimicrobial agents. *Journal of Infectious Diseases* 1985; 151:388–98.

Musher DM. Antibiotics: the medium is the message. *Reviews of Infectious Diseases* 1983; 5:809–12.

Smith MC. Drug product advertising and prescribing: a review of the evidence. *American Journal of Hospital Pharmacy* 1977; 34:1208–24.

Waud DR. Pharmaceutical promotions—a free lunch? *New England Journal of Medicine* 1992; 327:351–53.

Wilkes MS, Doblin BH, Shapiro MF. Pharmaceutical advertisements in leading medical journals: experts' assessments. *Annals of Internal Medicine* 1992; 116:912–19.

Yu VL, Stoehr GP, Starling RC, Shogan JE. Empiric antibiotic selection by physicians: evaluation of reasoning strategies. *American Journal of the Medical Sciences* 1991; 301:165–72.

Chapter 11. Fifteen Things You Can Do to Avert Catastrophe

Adams WG, Deaver KA, Cochi SL. Decline of childhood *Haemophilus influenzae* type b (Hib) disease in the Hib era. *Journal of the American Medical Association* 1993; 269:221–26.

Avorn J, Soumerai SB. Improving drug-therapy decisions through educational outreach. *New England Journal of Medicine* 1983; 308:1457–63.

Avorn J, Soumerai SB, Taylor W, et al. Reduction of incorrect antibiotic dosing through a structured educational order form. *Archives of Internal Medicine* 1988; 148:1720–24.

Doebbling BN, Stanley GL, Sheetz CT, et al. Comparative efficacy of alternative handwashing agents in reducing nosocomial infections in intensive care units. *New England Journal of Medicine* 1992; 327:88–93.

Fedson DS. Clinical practice and public policy for influenza and pneumococcal vaccination of the elderly. *Clinics in Geriatric Medicine* 1992; 8:183–99.

Gaynes RP, Culver DH, Emori TG, et al. The national nosocomial infections surveillance system: plans for the 1990s and beyond. *American Journal of Medicine* 1991; 91(supplement 3B):116S–120S.

Goldmann DA. Contemporary challenges for hospital epidemiology. *American Journal of Medicine* 1991; 91(supplement 3B):8S–14S.

Harvey KJ, Stewart R, Hemming M, et al. Educational antibiotic advertising. *Medical Journal of Australia* 1986; 145:28–31.

Himmelberg CJ, Pleasants RA, Weber DJ, et al. Use of antimicrobial drugs in adults before and after removal of a restriction policy. *American Journal of Hospital Pharmacy* 1991; 48:1220–27.

Kollisch, DO. Of mugs and marketing: the Robin Hood solution. *Journal of the American Medical Association* 1992; 267:55.

Kuntz ID. Structure-based strategies for drug design and discovery. *Science* 1992; 257:1078–82.

Landgren FT, Harvey KJ, Mashforn L, et al. Changing antibiotic prescribing by educational marketing. *Medical Journal of Australia* 1988; 149:595–99.

Mahan MJ, Slauch JM, Mekalanos JJ. Selection of bacterial virulence genes that are specifically induced in host tissues. *Science* 1993; 259:686–88.

Martone WJ. Year 2000 objectives for preventing nosocomial infections: how do we get there? *American Journal of Medicine* 1991; 91(supplement 3B):39S–43S.

McDonald PJ. Antibiotic guidelines—do we know where we're going? *Medical Journal of Australia* 1989; 150:610–11.

McGowan JE. New laboratory techniques for hospital infection control. *American Journal of Medicine* 1991; 91(supplement 3B):245S–250S.

Merz B. DNA probes promise to transform diagnosis of infectious disease. *Journal of the American Medical Association* 1987; 258:301–2.

Moleski RJ, Andriole VT. Role of the infectious disease specialist in containing costs of antibiotics in the hospital. *Reviews of Infectious Diseases* 1986; 8:488–93.

O'Brien TF. Global surveillance of antibiotic resistance. *New England Journal of Medicine* 1992; 326:339–40.

Ranki M. New microbial diagnosis. *Annals of Medicine* 23:381–88.

Rozenberg-Arska M, Visser MR. Infectious disease therapy in the 1990s: where are we heading? *Drugs* 1992; 43:629–36.

Schaffner W, Ray WA, Federspiel CF, Miller WO. Improving antibiotic prescribing in office practice. *Journal of the American Medical Association* 1983; 250:1728–32.

Shapiro ED, Berg AT, Austrian R, et al. The protective efficacy of polyvalent pneumococcal polysaccharide vaccine. *New England Journal of Medicine* 1991; 325:1453–60.

Shaw J. Antibiotic guidelines and antibiotic policies. *Medical Journal of Australia* 1983; 143:204–5.

Stone R. Déjà vu guides the way to new antimicrobial steroid. *Science* 1993; 259:1125.

Tompkins LS. The use of molecular methods in infectious diseases. *New England Journal of Medicine* 1992; 327:1290–97.

Towner KJ. Detection of antibiotic resistance genes with DNA probes. *Journal of Antimicrobial Chemotherapy* 1992; 30:1–2.

Vogels MTE, van der Meer JWM. Use of immune modulators in nonspecific therapy of bacterial infections. *Antimicrobial Agents and Chemotherapy* 1992; 36:1–5.

Weinstein RA, Kabins SA. Strategies for prevention and control of multiple drug-resistant nosocomial infection. *American Journal of Medicine* 1981; 70:449–54.

Wentz DK, Osteen AM, Canon MI. Continuing medical education: unabated debate. *Journal of the American Medical Association* 1992; 268:1118–19.

Yu VL, Fagan LM, Wraith SM, et al. Antimicrobial selection by a computer: a blinded evaluation by infectious disease experts. *Journal of the American Medical Association* 1979; 242:1279–82.

Index